Final MB

to Gillian and James

Final MB
A Guide to Success in Clinical Medicine

H. R. Dalton MB BS BSc MRCP

Foreword by
K. B. Saunders
Professor of Medicine, St George's Hospital Medical School, London

CHURCHILL LIVINGSTONE
EDINBURGH LONDON MELBOURNE AND NEW YORK 1991

CHURCHILL LIVINGSTONE
Medical Division of Longman Group UK Limited

Distributed in the United States of America by Churchill
Livingstone Inc., 650 Avenue of the Americas, New York,
N. Y. 10011 and by associated companies, branches and
representatives throughout the world.

First published 1991
  Reprinted 1993

ISBN 0-443-04376-0

British Library Cataloguing in Publication Data
Dalton, H. R.
  A guide to success in clinical medicine.
  1. Medicine. Diagnosis
  I. Title
  616.075

Library of Congress Cataloging in Publication Data
Dalton, H. R. (Harry Richard)
    Final M.B.: a guide to success in clinical medicine/
    H. R. Dalton
    foreword by K. B. Saunders.
       p.   cm.
    1. Internal medicine—Examinations, questions, etc.
    I. Title. [DNLM: 1. Clinical Medicine—examination
    questions. WB 18 D152f]
    RC58.D35   1991
    616'.0076 — dc20
    DNLM/DLC
    for Library of Congress
                                        90-1792
                                        CIP

The
publisher's
policy is to use
**paper manufactured
from sustainable forests**

Produced by Longman Singapore Publishers (Pte) Ltd
Printed in Singapore

Foreword

Passing finals is a question of doing simple things well. The process is mainly designed to detect the small percentage of students who are not ready to perform as house physicians or surgeons, so that they can be given further undergraduate training (and also to detect a small proportion of high-fliers). The ambition of any Dean or Professor of Medicine is to get a 100% pass rate, but we are almost always frustrated. This does not please us: it is no fun failing students and examining resits is a terrible bore.

If you are a passenger in a motor car, you can usually tell within a few minutes whether the driver is competent or not, though it would often be difficult to say precisely how. When an examiner watches a student examining an abdomen or using an ophthalmoscope, it is usually rapidly obvious whether the student is competent, regardless of their findings. You can 'miss the spleen' and still pass. Techniques of clinical examination need practising until they become automatic: when they do, and if they are done right, the practitioner looks competent.

There are, however, certain tricks of the trade handed down from generation to generation, which are worth knowing. They involve obvious things like dress, but also more subtle matters. These are well set out by Dr Dalton. There is also, whether examiners like it or not, a corpus of experience in the practical clinical field outside which the examination can rarely stray. You will see mitral stenosis, possibly for the first time. You won't see hypoglycaemic coma. Finally, there are questions or topics which come up frequently and are worth special revision.

Don't confuse this book with a textbook of medicine. Do use it as you would use revision ward rounds in the months before finals.

Dr Dalton is a highly regarded revision teacher and what he writes makes good sense. I don't agree with all of it, but then, I often pass students who say things I don't agree with, provided such points aren't too numerous, and are well argued.

London, 1991   K.B.S.

Preface

This book is intended primarily for final year medical students who are preparing for their final clinical examination in General Medicine.

It is not written as a complete textbook of medicine and should not be treated as such. It is very much an exam-orientated book, and is meant to alleviate some of the suffering of those nail-biting weeks just prior to the final MB.

It concentrates on the type of questions asked by the examiners and how to respond in a way which will give the candidate the best chance of success.

The majority of the book concentrates on the Short Cases, as from my experience students find these the most difficult. I have also included sections on the written paper, the Long Cases, and the viva, as I feel it is important to put the approach to the Short Cases in context.

At the end of Chapter 1 and Chapters 4–11, there is a 'key questions' section. This consists of some questions which are amongst the more frequently asked, and are included for you to consider. You will find many, but not all, of the answers in the main text. If you can't find the answer discuss it with your colleagues, or look it up in one of those big fat reference books.

Oxford, 1991   H.R.D.

Acknowledgements

I would like to thank the following for their help and advice, without whom this book would not have been possible:

Mr M. Birch (illustrations), Dr M. Hall (cartoons), Dr A. Wilson, Ms G. Adams, Dr I. Iheanacho, Dr N. J. Reynolds, Dr J. Turner, Dr A. Ndrika, Dr A. Mlcahy, Dr S. Choy, Dr A. Kohn, Ms G. E. A. Rainsberry (index).

I am greatly indebted to Mrs R. Lenham for typing the manuscript.

The colour photographs were very kindly sponsored by Pharmax, the manufacturers of Predfoam and Buccal Suscard.

I wish to thank Dr I. Iheanacho and Dr N. J. Reynolds for their help with editing and proofreading this book.

Oxford, 1991   H.R.D.

Contents

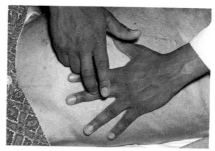

Plate 1 Percussing flank dullness (see Chapter 6).

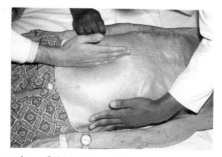

Plate 2 Demonstrating a fluid thrill (see Chapter 6).

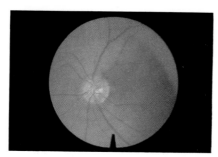

Plate 3 Fundoscopic appearance of diabetic retinopathy: new vessel formation (Chapter 10).

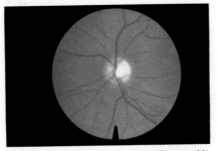

Plate 4 Fundoscopic appearance of optic atrophy (Chapter 10).

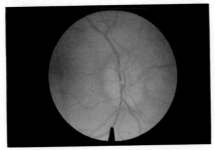

Plate 5 Fundoscopic appearance of papilloedema (Chapter 10).

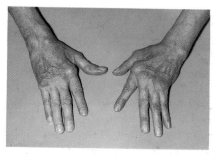

Plate 6a Rheumatoid arthritis. Note the prominent metacarpal heads (metacarpophalangeal subluxation), ulnar deviation of the fingers and wasting of the small muscles of the hand.

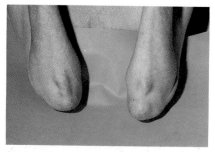

Plate 6b Rheumatoid nodules at the elbows.

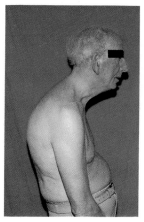

Plate 7 The typical 'question mark' posture of ankylosing spondylitis (Chapter 11).

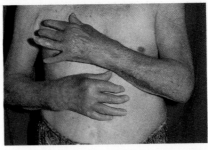

Plate 8a Psoriatic arthropathy: arthritis mutilans (Chapter 11). Note the patches of psoriasis at the elbows and deformity of the hands, including the distal interphalangeal joints.

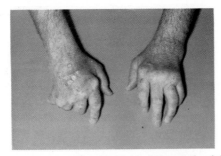

Plate 8b Another combination of psoriatic skin lesions and a deforming arthritis of the hands. This time the arthritis is due to rheumatoid arthritis (distal interphalangeal joints spared) and the psoriasis is an incidental finding.

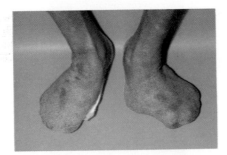

Plate 9 This shows some of the complications of diabetes affecting the lower limb (Chapters 8 and 12): bilateral toe amputations (peripheral arterial disease); Charcot ankle joint (peripheral neuropathy). You can just make out the edge of a dressing on the right: this covers an infected, painless ulcer on the sole of the foot.

General principles

1 The examination

The final MB examination varies at different medical schools. However, in general terms, there is always a written section and a clinical section.

(a) THE WRITTEN PAPER

Past papers are available and it is essential to get hold of these to see what you are up against. 'Question spotting' is notoriously inaccurate and not to be recommended, but practising your answering technique in both the multiple choice questions (MCQs) and essay section is definitely worthwhile. I would suggest that you ask one of your tutors (preferably someone who marks the real thing) to go over your model answers with you.

Most MCQs in medicine are marked in a sophisticated manner these days. The following scheme is used:

$+1$ = correct response.
-1 = incorrect response.
0 = no response.

In addition to this, questions are often graded as to the degree of difficulty, so that a correct answer to a difficult question carries relatively more weight than to an easy one. The trick is to try and answer the right number of questions (approximately 85–90% of the total), avoid wild guesses and try to avoid answering easy questions incorrectly. Admittedly this is easier said than done, but attempting past papers will help you gain more confidence. The written section is generally 'close marked' and so to miss out a question completely can be totally disastrous. Having said this, if it happens to you don't start sharpening up the bread knife! I have known several people do this, and still pass. You must practise your examination technique on the essay questions and pay particular attention to:

(1) Time allocation to each answer.
(2) Structure of the answer. Make it easier for the examiner to read and mark by setting it out in clearly headed sections.
(3) Legibility. It has been shown in several studies that answers written in good legible script gain better marks. You need to balance this against (1).
(4) Answering a question you know nothing about.

You may not realise it but there will be relatively few things you know absolutely nothing about. Most questions, you should, at least, have some vague idea about. I recommend leaving the question you know least about until last. Doing good answers to the other questions you know more about will give you confidence and a chance to mull over the grey area of your last question at the back of your mind.

When you come to put pen to paper for the final question, you may realise you know more about it than you at first thought. If you are still having trouble you could put the subject matter of the question through a 'sieve' and see what comes out at the other end. There are many such 'sieves' in local usage — I recommend my students make up their own, as these mnemonics are more easily remembered.

Whatever you do put *something* down on paper as your answer to that difficult question. A blank sheet will score 0 out of 10; an absolutely appallingly dreadful answer may score 3 out of 10. This is an enormous difference in a close-marked paper.

I will say no more about the written paper. Obviously it is essential to do the necessary book-work to pass, but I think attention to the above points will help a little knowledge go further.

(b) CLINICAL PAPER

The clinical section directly involves patients and is divided into two sections: 'long case' and the 'short cases'.

The clinical section is usually held in a purpose-built room, which comprises a number of clinical cubicles and some cubicles for the examiners.

The long case

Candidates are usually given 45 minutes to take a history from and examine a long case. In addition to this, 10 – 15 minutes are set aside for the candidate to explain the history and physical findings to the examiners. You may well be taken back to the patient to demonstrate the clinical signs that you have elicited.

Forty-five minutes may not seem a long time but, with practice under examination conditions, it is usually more than adequate. It is best to try to finish the case within 40 minutes so leaving a valuable 5 minutes' thinking time. This will give you a chance to gather your thoughts, and it will also give you an opportunity to decide which aspects of the case to bring out when you present the case to the examiners. I strongly recommend you use this time to summarise the case in *writing*. You should always write down the history and examination, in any case, as it is often helpful or necessary to refer to your notes during your presentation. At the end I recommend that you write five brief paragraphs (of 2–3 sentences each) in summary.

(1) Summary of the history.
(2) Summary of clinical findings.
(3) Differential diagnosis.
(4) Investigations you think necessary.
(5) Relevant treatment — both immediate and long-term.

The patients for the long case may be taken from the disciplines of general medicine, geriatric medicine, psychiatry or paediatrics. They are usually selected for the examination because of their ability to give a clear history. Occasionally a candidate may get a patient who, for one reason or another, cannot give a clear history. This may cause you to panic — but don't. Simply do the best you can with the conditions and explain to the examiners that you had difficulty taking a reliable history and the reasons for it. For example, the patient could be demented, have a malfunctioning hearing aid, or be dysarthric or unable to speak English. You might like to suggest to the examiners that you would like to demonstrate why the history was so difficult to obtain (they may not have realised this). This would involve, for example, doing an abbreviated mental test score on the patient, or the demonstration of dysarthria in a patient with a cerebellar syndrome. Try to build up a rapport with the patient — he may tell you what the diagnosis is. The 'professional patient' (i.e. one who is frequently called up for examinations) may even know what clinical signs he is supposed to have!

The patients are drawn from two sources. Firstly, there are the in-patients. These are patients who have been admitted as an emergency to hospital in the days prior to the examination. They will be in the recovery phase from their current illness. Sick patients should never be included in the examination. Current in-patients tend to be in a minority. This is simply a matter of logistics for the people organising the examination. There are usually not enough patients who are fit enough, able to give a good history, or have interesting clinical signs to go round.

The numbers are made up from out-patients who are brought in specially for the examination. These are people with (usually) chronic physical signs, who can give a good history. Most centres have a list of patients on whom they call, which is added to and subtracted from each year. Among their number will be 'professional patients' who have been used numerous times before. They are often the most helpful to candidates, for reasons already outlined.

Paediatric cases can be daunting. Trying to get a history from and examine an uncooperative child can be a nightmare. You *must* get the mother on your side. They are usually very well informed about the condition Little Johnny is suffering from. Enlist the mother's help in both the history and examination as much as possible. If all else fails you can always ask the mother what the diagnosis is and what treatment the patient is having — she may also know what the physical signs are.

Psychiatric cases are usually straightforward. You will know if you have a psychiatric long case because the registrar will usually tell you that a 'physical examination is unnecessary'. The case will either be depressed, manic or schizophrenic. Occasional cases of anorexia, bulimia, alcohol-related problems, obsessive/compulsive behaviour or personality disorder are included.

The long case history

It is important to ask the patient's name. I have heard of a candidate who went to see a long case and could find absolutely nothing wrong in the history or examination. He told the examiners this, and they duly took him back to the patient:

Table 1.1

Name:

Age:

Occupation:

Main complaint:

History of present complaint:

Past medical history:

Current medication:

Known allergies:

Family history:

Social history:

Systems review:

Examiner (to the patient): 'What is your name, sir?'
Patient (to examiner): 'Napoleon Bonaparte'

The history should be written down on paper as it is taken. Paper is provided. This should be done in the formalised traditional method which you have been taught since your first day on the wards. See Table 1.1.

When you present the history to the examiners do it in an intelligent way. Emphasise the positive and relevant negative findings in the history. You must go through each section in turn. Do not miss anything out.

These days the examiners are very keen on the social history — in other words how the patient's illness affects his/her daily life. You should find out all the details regarding Meals on Wheels, home helps, district nurse, social worker, steps at home, Zimmer frames, sticks, crutches, getting out of the house, day centres, which room the patient sleeps in, family, neighbours, care-givers, GP home visits, financial problems, etc., etc.

Examining the long case

You must perform a quick, but thorough, examination. You must, obviously, pay particular attention to the relevant areas indicated by your history: do not miss *anything* out. A generalised scheme for examination is set out in Table 1.2.

Present all the findings. Lay emphasis on positive findings and

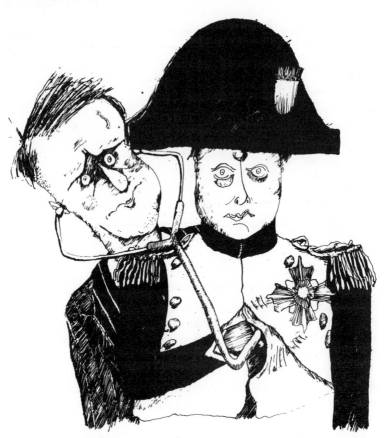

'*Not tonight, Josephine.*'

Table 1.2

General observation
Breasts
Thyroid
Skin
Evidence of jaundice, anaemia, cyanosis, clubbing, lymphadenopathy
Scars

Cardiovascular system
Pulse, blood pressure, JVP
Apex beat, heart sounds 1 and 2, additional sounds, murmurs
Thrill, heaves, palpable heart sounds
Peripheral pulses, peripheral oedema
Bruits
Retinae

Table 1.2 (*contd*)

Respiratory system
Respiratory rate (breaths per minute)
Trachea
Chest expansion
Percussion note
Breath sounds
Tactile vocal fremitus
Auditory resonance
Whispering pectoriloquy
Sputum pot

Abdomen
General observation: observation of abdomen for obvious fullness or mass
Signs of chronic liver disease
Tenderness, rebound?, guarding?
Masses
Organs
  liver
  kidneys
  spleen
  bladder
  gravid uterus
Hernial orifices
Bowel sounds

Do not examine the genitalia or do a PR, but express the desirability of doing so

Central nervous system
Orientation
  time
  place
  person
Cranial nerves I–XII
Tone
Power
Reflexes
Sensation
  light touch
  pain
  joint position sense
  vibration sense
Gait
Cerebellar signs
Don't forget the jaw jerk, and Romberg's sign
There is a lot to get through in the time allocated. A detailed neurological examination should be done, but clearly if time is a problem and no neurological pathology is indicated by the history, it would probably be necessary to curtail this to a brief version.
Do not forget to take the blood pressure, look in the sputum pot and look for clues left by examiners, for example temperature chart or diabetic drinks on the locker. If there is a sample of the patient's urine, test it. If there is no urine testing kit ask for it, or tell the examiners that none was available.

relevant negative findings. If you could find no abnormality at all, say so (at the start).

The last few minutes of your time with your long case should be spent summarising the case in writing, as already discussed. I cannot emphasise enough the importance of these last few minutes for gathering your thoughts. It will be the one chance for you to think about what *you* would like to talk about to the examiners regarding the case you have seen. If possible you should try to steer the examiners in this direction, so that you are in an area you know something about.

The examiners

They expect candidates to give a concise, thorough and intelligent account of the case they have seen, presented in a formal way, as explained. The examiner will tell you if he wants something else.

Occasionally they will stop you in full stream or start off by asking you a question. You should be prepared to answer questions such as:

(1) What is the differential diagnosis?
(2) What tests would you order?
(3) What do you think about the patient's treatment?
(4) How would you have managed this patient in casualty?

I will say more about the examiners in a later chapter.

Practice

See as many long cases as you can to practise your technique. Present cases to each other, and to the houseman, registrar, consultant: in fact anybody you can get to listen. Get them to criticise you constructively. Think about their criticisms.

Some people have great difficulty communicating verbally, particularly under stress. I recommend that if you are such a candidate you get a dictaphone and practise presenting the case to the machine. Play it back and listen to what you sound like. Remember that the machine does not lie. Keep on practising until you are perfect.

The short cases

Approximately 15 minutes are set aside for you to be examined on short cases. These are usually general medicine or paediatrics. If you saw a paediatric long case you will often get general medicine short cases and vice versa.

The examiners will tell you exactly what they want you to do and you should follow their instructions implicitly. For example, 'examine this praecordium' means look at, palpate and auscultate the chest wall which overlies the heart. Do exactly that.

'Examine the heart' means do a full examination of the cardiovascular system starting at the hands (see later chapter).

The examiners will then ask you questions such as:

'What is the diagnosis?'
'What did you think of this murmur?'
'What abnormality did you find?'

This is often followed up by the question:

'What are the causes of X', or
'What are the associations of X?'

It is therefore essential to have a brief list of the causes of any sign or clinical diagnosis. The list should be brief and should include the most common causes first. It is important that these lists are not too long so they are easily at your fingertips. I will say more about this in the later parts of this book.

In psychiatric short cases you must be prepared to do a brief mental state examination on the patient. Alternatively, an increasingly popular way of testing candidates' ability to assess a mental state is by means of video recording. A video is shown of a patient's mental state being assessed. You will then be asked to comment on what you have seen.

The short cases give the examiners an unique chance to see what you are like in a clinical setting. One of the things they are looking for is a professional examination. This can be hard to project under such intense pressure, unless you are on 'automatic pilot'.

The concept of being on 'automatic pilot' is a simple one. You need to practise your examination technique in a pressure setting, preferably with a senior doctor watching. Practise examining any system, organ or anatomical region you can think of. Practise it again and again (under pressure). Eventually you will achieve the dizzy heights of being on 'automatic pilot'. That is, you will not need to think about what bit to examine next (when you are asked to examine a respiratory system for example) because you will do it automatically. You are now free to think about other things during the examination, such as making it look stylish and professional, what are the physical signs, what is the diagnosis, etc.

The examiners will also want to see that you are conventional, competent and have common sense and a caring attitude. Always be polite to the patient. Never hurt the patient. Always make sure he is comfortable. The short cases hold terror for some because you are really on the spot. The patient is in front of you and the examiners want to know the answers. You have little time to think about what you are going to say. It is possible to gain a vital few seconds thinking time in two ways during the short cases.

Firstly, when you are using your stethoscope. You can use this period for extra thinking time. You will have heard the necessary physical signs — you just need a few seconds to think. Leave the stethoscope in position (appearing to be examining) but all the while you have an extra few seconds to gather your thoughts on the case in front of you.

Secondly, help the patient to get comfortable after you have finished examining him (for example help him on with his dressing gown). This not only gives an extra second or two's thinking time, but presents a caring attitute to the examiners — they will like it!

I cannot overemphasise the importance of the need to practise. Get a doctor to take a small group of you to see some model short cases prior to the exam. Encourage mutual (constructive) criticism. Practise and practise again. Once you are on 'automatic pilot' there will be no looking back.

The viva

At the end of the examination you have the viva voce. This entails approximately a 10-minute interview with two examiners. In the final MB viva the examiners can be from any field of general medicine or the allied specialties of paediatrics, psychiatry, community medicine, dermatology, geriatrics, etc. They are free to take any line of questioning they like. General physicians tend to concentrate on questions regarding the emergency management of patients.

Example 1

'How do you manage acute myocardial infarction?'

You should concentrate on the following areas: history; examination; special investigations; treatment.

History. Classically the patient complains of crushing central chest pain radiating down the left arm, associated with nausea and sweating. Remember patients may have atypical stories, and myocardial infarction can present in many different ways.

Examination. Clinical examination may be unremarkable. Remember to say you would look for signs of left ventricular dysfunction (e.g. third heart sound, crackles at the bases, hypotension). Look for signs which may give a clue to the 'risk factors' for ischaemic heart disease, e.g. nicotine-stained fingers, xanthelasmata, etc.

Special investigations. Those you would need in this situation are an ECG, a chest X-ray, urea and electrolytes, serial ECGs and serial cardiac enzymes. It is important to emphasise the practical aspects of managing such a case. You should mention that you would do a quick assessment of the patient in casualty, have a look at the ECG and chest X-ray, and on the basis of this institute management straight away. Do not forget to mention pain relief. This is most important. An intravenous injection of diamorphine together with prochlorperazine is mandatory to relieve the patient's pain. Modern management of acute myocardial infarction includes infusion of streptokinase (given in the casualty department) and aspirin. It is important to know what the patient's potassium level is. Post-myocardial infarct cardiac arrhythmias are least common when the patient's potassium is in the range of 4–4.5 mmol/l. You should mention that the patient should be transferred as soon as possible to a coronary care bed, where monitoring facilities and nursing expertise are available. Do not forget to mention the nursing aspects of the case and the stepped programme of rehabilitation in the recovery phase. Most centres would agree that a patient who has received streptokinase following acute myocardial infarction should have an exercise test prior to discharge.

Example 2

'How would you assess the severity and initiate treatment in a patient with acute severe asthma?'

Again you ought to consider the history, examination, special investigations and treatment.

History. This may be difficult to obtain from the patient. If the patient is so breathless as to be unable to speak in sentences, that patient will have severe asthma. The past history is important — ask about the pattern of past attacks (e.g. history of requiring mechanical ventilation, speed of onset of symptoms, number of hospital admissions, etc.).

Examination. Assessing the severity of acute severe asthma is sometimes quite difficult. It is most important to determine whether the patient's asthma falls into the mild, moderate or severe category: it will influence your management greatly. The parameters you should look for which indicate that the patient has acute severe asthma are:

(1) Sinus tachycardia greater than 100 beats per minute.
(2) Inability to speak in sentences.
(3) Cyanosis.
(4) Pulsus paradoxus (greater than 20 mmHg).
(5) Silent chest (the asthma is so severe the patient is unable to get enough air in and out of the chest to create a wheeze).
(6) Peak flow. This needs to be related to the patient's normal measurement. A peak flow of 100 in a patient with a normal peak flow of 600 indicates very severe asthma. On the other hand, someone with a normal peak flow of 200 (who suffers with chronic asthma) who has a peak flow of 100 may only have a mild or moderate attack.

Investigations. Blood gases are an essential investigation; a falling Po_2 and a rising Pco_2 carries important implications. A chest X-ray is mandatory to exclude a pneumothorax, which occasionally occurs in severe asthma.

Treatment. In the treatment section you should include the use of 100% oxygen, regular nebulised bronchodilators, physiotherapy, intravenous corticosteroids, intravenous antibiotics (if indicated), intravenous aminophylline (omit the loading dose if the patient is already on theophylline derivatives), monitor the patient with an ECG monitor and serum theophylline levels. Patients with very severe asthma unresponsive to the above treatment and deteriorating may well need ventilation.

Example 3

'How would you manage a paracetamol overdose?'

Again history, examination and special investigations are important.

History. This is vitally important. You may need to question relatives, friends, psychiatric workers, etc. Ambulancemen may bring empty bottles of tablets or a suicide note.

Examination. This may be normal, but if it is a multiple over-dose, including paracetamol, the patient may be drowsy, e.g. if they have taken large amounts of hypnotics or alcohol in addition to the paracetamol.

Special investigations. These include baseline clotting studies, baseline liver function tests and a serum paracetamol level. As you will be aware, there is a graph which shows paracetamol levels against time on which there is a treatment line. If the patient is near this treatment line or above it for a specified time (which is always greater than 4 hours) the patient will require treatment with intravenous acetylcysteine as per the BNF. You should mention that you would ring up the local poisons unit for further expert advice.

In patients who have taken a serious overdose of paracetamol more than 24 hours previously treatment with acetylcysteine is ineffective. These patients are at risk of gross hepatocellular necrosis and should be monitored closely with serial prothrombin times and liver function tests. They may well require referral to a regional liver unit for further, more specialised, treatment.

Occasionally examiners may ask questions relating to articles which have been in the popular press or medical journals. It is worth while having a look through recent copies of the *BMJ* and *Lancet* prior to your viva. Keep a vague eye out for medical articles in the newspapers and on TV.

In summary, in the viva you need to show the examiners that you have common sense and an adequate range of medical knowledge. They will be trying to find out if you have spent any time in casualty and seen treatment of emergency cases. They will also try to find out that you are up to date with current medical thinking. If you know nothing about a subject on which they are asking you questions you should tell the examiner this. More than likely he will move onto something else. Remember that they are trying to pass rather than fail you.

KEY QUESTIONS

The 20 questions below are samples of viva voce questions which students have been asked in the past.

You will notice that some of the questions are particularly difficult or vague (marked +). If you get one of these do not worry — you are either honours material, or the examiner knows you have already passed and is just amusing himself. If you get a simple question, now that is a different matter.

(1) What advice would you give a 55-year-old male who had an uncomplicated myocardial infarction 10 days ago?

(2) What is the natural history of aortic stenosis?

(3) What is the treatment of tension pneumothorax?

(4) How would you treat an asymptomatic 80-year-old female with blood pressure of 170/110?

(5) What are the implications for the future of medical care delivery of the Government's recent White Paper? (+)

(6) What antibiotic therapy would you start (before microbiological confirmation is available) for a fit 25-year-old male with a primary community-acquired chest infection?

(7) What are the causes of upper gastrointestinal haemorrhage?

(8) What are the non-pharmacological means of therapy and support which are available for patients with HIV-associated disease? How could these be improved? (+)

(9) What is a Sengstaken tube?

(10) Define anaemia.

(11) How would you assess the control of a diabetic in out-patients?

(12) How would you manage a 40-year-old female with bloody diarrhoea?

(13) How would you manage an 18-year-old female patient who is deeply unconscious in the casualty department?

(14) Tell me about 'zoonoses' and their relationship to the Channel Tunnel. (+)

(15) A man falls down in front of you in the bus queue. He has no pulse and is not breathing. Describe the next 10 minutes in detail.

(16) What are the medical risks of the combined oral contraceptive?

(17) What is an NMR scan? What are the indications for an NMR scan at present in the UK? Where is the nearest NMR scanner situated? (+)

(18) How would you manage a 65-year-old male patient (in the casualty department) with severe, persistent central chest pain?

(19) What is a macule? Name some conditions in which they are found.

(20) Who was Dupytren? What is the significance of his sign?

2 Examiners and the candidate

THE EXAMINERS

The clinical examiners traditionally work in pairs. If the examination paper is an 'internal' one there will be one examiner from your teaching hospital group and one examiner who has been invited from outside. If the examination is 'external' both examiners will be alien to your previous experience.

You are usually told several days in advance who your examiners are and where they are from. It is helpful to find out a little about them, particularly if they have any 'foibles'. Some examiners have particular ways they like the abdomen examined, for example. If you know any students from the medical school at which the examiner works it is well worth a 10p phone call to find out such information in advance. Check with candidates from your own medical school from previous years, as they may have met them in the exam setting and could possibly give you valuable tips.

You must remember that the examiners may have to examine for 4 or 5 days. They are human (believe it or not) and are subject to feelings of hunger, boredom and irritability like the rest of us. This should not affect you in any serious way. However, if you are ever in the position of being the registrar who organises the examination, please make sure the mid-morning coffee and biscuits arrive on time, or you may find yourself looking for another job!

Individual medical school pass rates are, in general, remarkably constant from year to year. The reason for this is not hard to discern: if they were to fail 30% of candidates one year and only 10% of candidates the next year this would create havoc in the employment market place. One year there would be not enough newly qualified doctors to fill the available house physician/surgeon posts, the next year there would be a glut of new doctors with consequent medical unemployment. The first scenario would not be popular with our senior medical colleagues, who would be at sea without a houseman. The second would not be popular with Her Majesty's Government, who are uneasy about unemployment at the best of times:

'New docs draw dole'.

Having said that the pass rate varies little from year to year, there are occasional hiccoughs when considerably more students fail than in previous years. The reasons for this are not entirely clear. It seems difficult to believe that the overall standard of candidate would vary much from year to year, especially in schools which have over 100 students per year. It is possible that the reasons for such discrepancies lie with the 'rogue examiner' who insists in failing more candidates than usual. Such examiners could be 'external' ('these X students are useless compared to my Y students') or 'internal' (e.g. a new head of department wanting either to stamp his authority on his new medical school or to teach the students a lesson they will not forget 'for not turning up to my teaching sessions').

THE CANDIDATE AND WHAT THE EXAMINERS ARE LOOKING FOR

In the final MB examination the examiners are trying to pass you (as opposed to trying to fail you, which is the situation in most postgraduate examinations). The attributes which the examiner are looking for are those which make a good house doctor and can be summarised by the three Cs.

(1) competence (and common sense).
(2) caring.
(3) conventionality.

Any serious deviation from these three attributes would result in the candidate being invited to reattend in 6 months' time.

Competence

The candidate must create the impression that he is used to being with patients; that he can do a quick, thorough examination (which looks professional); and that he can talk in common sense terms about his findings.

Caring

The candidate must demonstrate a caring attitude to his *patients* during the examination. Never hurt the patient. *Always* ask the patient if he is comfortable. Introduce yourself to the patient at the start, and ask permission to examine the relevant part or parts. You will be under intense stress during the examination, but remember that the patient has feelings too; *never* put the patient in an embarrassing position.

Conventionality

You must appear to be conventional, even if you are not. Men should wear a conventional suit in blue or grey, white shirt, plain tie and black shoes. Hair should be short but conservative. Women should wear a smart dress or a two piece, nothing too revealing or outrageous. Attitudes should be conventional. Always call the patient by his name: Mr X or Mrs Y. Try to smile and be confident. Do not be overconfident. Examiners do not like this, and with good reasons. Do not try to tell jokes or be too jovial.

On no account must you argue with the examiner — even if you know you are right. Examiners regard this as insulting. More importantly, they will probably fail you. Such overconfidence is thought of in a poor light. The reason for this is that when housemen are overconfident and unaware of their personal professional limitations they seriously jeopardise the health of their patients: this may cause unnecessary suffering and possibly death. Examiners, therefore, often fail overconfident candidates, and this usually comes as a nasty shock to the person involved.

In summary, you have to give the examiner the impression that, if his mother were ill, he would not mind you being the doctor looking after her.

3 Equipment

MIND AND BODY

The most important piece of equipment is yourself: your mind and body must be sharp and in good working order on the big day. It is up to you to make sure that this is the case.

Do not stay up all night before the day of the examination learning the 25 causes of atrial fibrillation, as you will be in no fit state to remember them in the high-pressure setting of the examination room. Get an early night if you can. A tot of whisky may help you sleep. I do not recommend any other kind of hypnotic.

A few candidates go to extreme lengths during the run up to the examinations. Some stay up all night trying to cram in those extra facts, filling themselves with endless cups of strong coffee. This is not recommended. Try to appreciate the difference between the time spent revising when you are alert and when you are not. A good hour's work when your mind is sharp is worth at least three when you are overtired with caffeine toxicity.

One or two candidates get so wound up by feelings of impending doom that they resort to pharmacological manipulations to try to improve their performance during the revision period, or the examination itself. I cannot stress how important it is to avoid this. It is a recipe for disaster. If you are in this position you ought to go and see someone you trust (preferably a doctor), *now*. Drugs which have been used are caffeine-based stimulants (to keep awake to revise), hypnotics (to sleep after a hard day's revising) and beta-blockers (to keep calm).

All of the above drugs have central nervous system effects and will impair your mental agility on the day. Do not take them. A couple of drinks at 10.30 p.m. in the local pub with colleagues after a hard day's revision is much kinder on the central nervous system, and infinitely more pleasant.

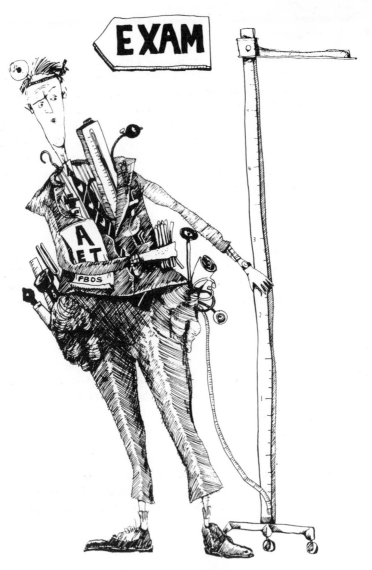

'Oh dear, I think I've forgotten my cotton wool balls.'

EQUIPMENT TO TAKE WITH YOU

Stethoscope

You should take your own stethoscope with you. This should be an ordinary one. If you bring out a £100 Littman Cardiology or St George's device the examiners may expect you to be able to hear the really difficult murmurs. This is called asking for trouble.

You need to check that it works properly before the exam. A contemporary of mine had the ear pieces of his stethoscope blocked up as a practical joke (by so-called 'friends') prior to his clinical finals! He could not hear a thing through it during the exam, but luckily he still managed to pass.

Ophthalmoscope

You ought to take your own, for several reasons. If you have not got one don't worry, one will be provided. Ophthalmoscopes vary in design; it is important to get to know yours before the exam. Get to know which knobs do what, make sure the batteries are new and the lenses are clean.

Neurological equipment

This will be provided at the examination. It is probably worth having some simple sensory testing equipment such as:

(1)   *Throw away* pins (HIV risk).
(2)   Cotton wool ball.
(3)   Tape measure.

These will not take up much room in your pockets.

Tuning forks, patella hammers, smell bottles, Snellen charts, etc., are best left for the medical school to provide, as they are rather bulky items.

Approach to the cases

This section of the book deals with the questions frequently asked by examiners, particularly in the short cases. The information given will also be applicable to the long cases, but is designed primarily to assist your approach to the short cases.

I have emphasised the cases which frequently crop up in the final clinical MB examination, but I have also briefly mentioned the rarer, more complicated, cases which appear occasionally.

4 The cardiovascular system (CVS)

THE TYPES OF QUESTIONS ASKED

You will be asked to do one of five things. Do exactly what the examiner asks you to.

(i) 'Examine the CVS'

This implies a full examination of the CVS. The patient should be comfortable on pillows at 45°. Introduce yourself to the patient and ask him if you may examine him. You should start at the hands and work your way up the arms to the face. Then examine the carotid pulse and JVP and then the heart. Do not forget to listen to the bases, feel for a liver edge, and abdominal aortic aneurysm. Feel all the peripheral pulses and for peripheral oedema. Do not forget to listen for bruits (including renal artery) and to feel for radiofemoral delay.

Follow the scheme set out in Table 4.1.

(ii) 'Examine the heart'

You should do exactly the same as in (i), starting at the hands. The examiner may stop you and tell you just to listen to the heart, but at least you have demonstrated that you are aware that the examination of the heart starts at the hands.

(iii) 'Auscultate the heart'

Do exactly what you have been told. Forget the hands and peripheral stuff and get your stethoscope plugged in.

Table 4.1   Scheme for examination of the CVS

General inspection
Hands
   peripheral cyanosis
   pallor
   clubbing (cyanotic congenital heart disease)
   splinters (infective endocarditis)
   nailfold infarction
   Quincke's sign (capillary pulsation of the nail beds found in aortic
   incompetence)
Radial pulse (make sure you time it with the second hand of your watch and
examine both pulses)
   rate
   rhythm
   character
Radiofemoral delay — coarctation of aorta
Blood pressure
Conjunctivae — anaemia
Mouth — mucosal membranes, central cyanosis or pallor
Carotid pulses (both) — but not at the same time

JVP
Make sure you examine the *internal* jugular vein. The patient's neck must be
relaxed. Remember the hepatojugular reflex. If you can't see the top of the JVP,
sit the patient up to 90°. Earlobes will waggle if the JVP is very high.

Look at the precordium
Scars (previous surgery)
Visible pulsations

Apex beat
Position: you must be seen to assess the exact position in terms of its relationship to
the intercostal space (from the angle of Louis) and the mid-clavicular line
   Quality diffuse (LV dilatation)
   thrusting (LV hypertrophy)
   dyskinetic segment (LV aneurysm)

Palpate precordium
Thrills (palpable murmurs): this is best done over each valvular area with the
   palm of the hand. The metacarpal heads seem to be the most sensitive area of
   the hand to use for this
Palpable heart sounds: for all intents and purposes this means feel for the first
   heart sound of mitral stenosis, which is frequently palpable. It is this which
   gives the apex beat its 'tapping' quality in this condition (difficult sign)
Auscultation
   murmurs
   third and fourth heart sounds
     Listen over each valvular area in turn with both the bell and diaphragm. Do
not forget to turn the patient into the left lateral position and listen to the apex
and axilla for mitral murmurs. Always sit the patient forwards and listen in
expiration to the aortic area and down the left sternal edge for the murmur of
aortic incompetence. Whilst in this position listen for carotid radiation/carotid
bruits.

Table 4.1 (*contd*)

Both bases
The patient is now sitting up. Take the opportunity to listen to both lung bases for crackles (left ventricular failure)

Abdomen
Liver, pulsatile (tricuspid regurgitation?)
Abdominal aortic aneurysm
Renal artery bruits
Peripheral pulses — examine all of them
Peripheral oedema, pitting?
Auscultate for bruits over the femorals and renal arteries. Do not forget to listen for carotid bruits

(iv) 'Examine the pulse'

You will usually be offered the right radial. If it is difficult to feel go to the left radial or carotid. Time the pulse with the second hand of your watch.

When examining the carotid pulse, do the right carotid artery with the left thumb and the left carotid artery with the right thumb.

The following parameters must be assessed when examining a pulse:

Rate.
Rhythm.
Character
slow rising (aortic stenosis)
water hammer (aortic regurgitation)
bisferiens (the double-topped pulse found in mixed aortic valve disease).

Occasionally the carotid pulse is visible from the end of the bed in aortic regurgitation (Corrigan's sign). In very severe aortic regurgitation the head may actually nod. This is called De Musset's sign.

(v) 'Examine the JVP'

The patient must be 45° with the head tilted to relax the strap muscles of the neck. It is usually best to turn the patient's face towards the left to achieve this. The JVP is best assessed in natural light; this may not be possible in the examination setting. It is essential to assess the internal jugular vein, not the external jugular. The external jugular vein may be raised due to local entrapment in the neck as it passes through the strap muscles and must therefore not be used as an indicator of the jugular venous pressure.

You need to know how to differentiate the JVP from carotid pulsation. The features to look for are:

(1) Double impulse in venous pulsation (not present in atrial fibrillation).
(2) The JVP falls on sitting up (usually). Carotid pulsation will not.
(3) Hepatojugular reflex. Venous return can be increased by pressing on the liver area. This will cause pulsation in the neck due to the JVP becoming more prominent. This distinguishes it from carotid pulsation.
(4) Filling from above. The JVP will fill from above when the internal jugular vein is pressed on firmly. Carotid pulsation will not.
(5) JVP is usually impalpable; the carotid pulsation is usually palpable.
(6) Level of pulsation in JVP usually falls in inspiration.

A raised JVP may be found in many conditions, but the common ones found in the examination are:

Left ventricular failure.
Severe right ventricular failure with tricuspid regurgitation. This may be secondary to valvular heart disease, ischaemic heart disease or cor pulmonale.

TYPICAL CASES

Cardiovascular short cases are common. This is because valvular heart disease is common (although now becoming less so) and the signs are chronic.

(1) Murmurs* (see Table 4.2)

(2) Right-sided murmurs‡

Tricuspid regurgitation.
Pulmonary stenosis.
Pulmonary incompetence.
Tricuspid stenosis.

Most people regard these as postgraduate murmurs.

---

* Very common.
† Common.
‡ Rare and/or difficult.

Table 4.2 Common MB murmurs

Murmur	Sign	Associated findings	Causes
Aortic stenosis	Ejection systolic murmur which radiates to carotids	Slow rising pulse Heaving apex Low systolic BP LVH on ECG and CXR	Congenital (bifid valve) Rheumatic
Aortic incompetence (regurgitation)	Blowing early diastolic murmur (aortic area or LSE with patient sitting up in expiration)	Water-hammer pulse Wide pulse pressure Corrigan's sign De Musset's sign Quincke's sign Heaving apex LVH on ECG and CXR	Rheumatic Dissecting aortic aneurysm Ankylosing spondylitis Marfan's syndrome Congenital, syphilis
Mitral stenosis	Rumbling mid-diastolic murmur at apex	Palpable first heart sound Presystolic accentuation if patient in sinus rhythm AF Opening snap	Usually rheumatic
Mitral incompetence	Pansystolic murmur at apex	Radiates to axilla best heard left lateral position	Rheumatic/LV dilatation (any cause) Ruptured chordae etc.

NB: *Aortic sclerosis* has exactly the same murmur as *aortic stenosis*, but none of the associated physical findings. It is due to thickening of the aortic valve (calcific age-related change) and is of no import, save that it has to be distinguished from aortic stenosis.

(3) Ventricular septal defect (VSD)‡

Rare. Sounds like mitral regurgitation at the left sternal edge (pan-systolic, harsh).

Causes
  congenital (maladie de Roger)
  post-MI (septal rupture — this is very rare in an exam as the patients are too sick).

(4) Atrial septal defect (ASD)‡

Rare. Fixed splitting of first heart sound with a pulmonary systolic flow murmur. (Postgraduate murmur).

  Cause
    congenital.

(5) Ischaemic heart disease★

Common long case (angina or post-myocardial infarction). Uncommon short case. History very important:

Cardiac pain.
Past medical history of hypertension, diabetes or hyperlipidaemia.
Family history.
Smoking.

  The patient may have no signs but look for xanthelasmata, hypertension, signs of diabetes, signs of left ventricular dysfunction.
  The ECG may be normal.

(6) Atrial fibrillation★

Very common.

Irregularly irregular pulse.
No 'a' waves in JVP (distinguishes it from multiple VEs, which can also cause an irregularly irregular pulse).
ECG shows irregular QRS complex with no 'P' waves.

Causes
  ischaemic heart disease★
  post myocardial infarction★
  mitral stenosis★
  thyrotoxicosis

pulmonary embolism
ASD
hypertensive heart disease
malignant infiltration of pericardium.

(7) Left ventricular failure

Although this is a very common diagnosis in everyday clinical practice, it is not often included in the examination. The reason for this is that patients with acute left ventricular failure are too unwell to be included. You may get someone in the recovery phase, but by this stage the signs will be disappearing or have gone altogether.

Signs
    tachypnoea
    central cyanosis
    sinus tachycardia
    raised JVP
    third heart sound
    crackles at both bases.

ECG shows left ventricular strain pattern.
CXR shows cardiomegaly, upper lobe blood diversion, interstitial shadowing, Kerley B lines, bat's wing appearance.

NB: These radiological signs can sometimes be strikingly unilateral.

(8) Hypertension*

Common long case.

Ninety percent primary*.
Ten percent secondary to
    renal disease*
    coarctation‡
    Cushing's disease‡
    Conn's syndrome‡
    acromegaly‡
    phaeochromocytoma‡.

Look for the effects of hypertension on the:

Eyes
    a-v nipping

    increased vessel tortuosity
    haemorrhage
    exudates
    papilloedema.
Heart — signs of LVH, ischaemic heart disease.
Kidneys — signs of chronic renal failure.
Peripheral vasculature.

You need to know a little bit about the investigations and the treatment of hypertension. These are commonly asked questions.

(9) Coarctation of the aorta‡

This is a very rare cause of hypertension. The signs to look for are:

(1) Radio-femoral delay.
(2) You can sometimes hear odd murmurs on the upper chest and back due to blood flow through the collaterals.
(3) Hypertension in the arms, hypotension in the legs.
(4) CXR
    rib notching
    post-stenotic dilatation of aorta.

(10) Situs invertus/dextrocardia‡

This is very very rare, but much loved by the examiners. Dextrocardia is one of the few causes of inaudible heart sounds. Other causes are:

Obesity*.
Chronic obstructive airways disease*.
Left pleural effusion (large)†.
Pericardial effusion‡.
Stethoscope not adjusted properly*.

If you think your patient has dextrocardia, other organs could also be transposed. There is an association with Kartaganer's syndrome.

(11) Aortic aneurysm

Abdominal — this is really a surgical case.
Thoracic‡ — the patient will complain of back and chest pain or a hoarse voice; signs include a tracheal tug and aortic regurgitation.

Causes
   syphilis‡
   atheroma†
   post dissection of aorta‡
   traumatic†.

KEY QUESTIONS

(1)   What are the causes of
    (i)   atrial fibrillation?
    (ii)   sinus tachycardia?
    (iii)   sinus bradycardia?
    (iv)   a raised JVP?
    (v)   aortic regurgitation?
    (vi)   aortic stenosis?
    (vii)   mitral regurgitation?
    (viii)   mitral stenosis?
    (ix)   left ventricular failure?
    (x)   an impalpable apex?
    (xi)   hypertension?
(2)   What are the risk factors associated with ischaemic heart disease?
(3)   How can you tell the difference clinically between
    (i)   a raised JVP and a visible carotid pulsation?
    (ii)   the murmur of aortic regurgitation and mitral stenosis?
    (iii)   the murmur of mitral regurgitation and aortic stenosis?
    (iv)   aortic stenosis and aortic sclerosis?

5 The respiratory system

The standard question in the short cases is to 'examine this patient's chest/respiratory system'. This should be done quickly but professionally. The patient should be comfortable, propped up by pillows at 45°. Introduce yourself. Ask permission to examine the patient. The guide for examination of the respiratory system is set out in Table 5.1.

TYPICAL CASES

(1) Clubbing★

Very common short case.

Causes
1. familial
2. idiopathic
3. carcinoma of the bronchus
   chronic suppurative lung disease
4. cystic fibrosis
5. empyema
6. bronchiectasis
7. lung abscess
8. fibrosing alveolitis
9. congenital cyanotic heart disease
10. infective endocarditis   14 Gastric Ca.
11. cirrhosis of liver‡
12. ulcerative colitis‡
13. Crohn's disease‡.   15 Coeliac disease   16 (TB)

You *must* know this list.

(2) Carcinoma of lung★

Very common case.

Table 5.1

General inspection
Respiratory rate
Hands
   clubbing (bronchial carcinoma)
   nicotine staining (COAD, bronchial carcinoma)
   CO_2 retention flap (respiratory failure)
   essential tremor ($\beta_2$agonist therapy)
   peripheral cyanosis
Pulse
Conjunctivae — suffusion (polycythaemia in COAD, or SVC obstruction)
Anaemia
Mucosae of mouth — central cyanosis
Trachea position — think of things which push (pleural effusion) or pull
(collapse) to one side
Nodes
   supraclavicular
   cervical
   occipital
   axillary

Supraclavicular nodes are best felt from behind to allow the fingertips to get
right in behind the clavicles

JVP
Raised in cor pulmonale and SVC obstruction

Apex beat
Determine the position exactly. This will, together with the tracheal position,
allow you to determine if there is any mediastinal shift

If the apex beat is impalpable, this is also useful information (see Chapter 4),
e.g. COAD

Right ventricular heave
Cor pulmonale

Expansion
This is arguably the most important sign in chest medicine. It is done quite
badly and is quite tricky to do well. Get an experienced doctor to show you
how. It tells you where the pathology is (pathology = side with least expansion).
It is bilaterally decreased in COAD

Percussion.
Auscultation.   } Compare right with
Tactile vocal fremitus.   } left on front of
Auditory resonance.   } chest.

Now you need to sit the patient forward and repeat the above examination
from 'expansion' on the back of the chest.

Whispering pectoriloquy
This is an over-rated clinical sign. The way to elicit it is to get the patient to
whisper 'one, one, one'. The sounds are heard better over an area of
consolidation or the top of a pleural effusion

Table 5.1   *(contd)*

Examine the ankles for pitting oedema (cor pulmonale?)

Sputum pot
Do not forget to look for it. It may give an important clue to the diagnosis, e.g. haemoptysis

CXR
Ask to see it

Look for:

  cachexia
  clubbing
  nicotine-stained fingers
  lymph nodes
  signs of intrathoracic involvement, for example:
    pleural effusion
    collapse
    recurrent chest infections.

Ask to see the chest X-ray and sputum pot.

Remember Pancoast's tumour. This is a carcinoma of the bronchus at the apex causing an ipsilateral Horner's syndrome (involvement of sympathetic chain) and ipsilateral wasting of the small muscles of the hand (T1 root of brachial plexus involved).

(3) Chronic obstructive airways disease★

Common case.

Signs
  nicotine-stained fingers
  CO_2 retention flap (rare in the exam)
  β_2 agonist tremor
  tachypnoea
  pursed lip breathing   } 'pink puffer'
  using accessory muscles of respiration

★ Very common.
† Common.
‡ Rare and/or difficult.

centrally cyanosed $\Big\}$ 'blue bloater'
peripheral oedema
overexpansion of the chest
barrel-shaped chest
hyperresonant percussion note
loss of cardiac dullness
impalpable apex beat
distant heart sounds
wheeze/reduced air entry.

You need to know about the aetiology, treatment and chest X-ray appearance. Patients have an obstructive deficit on respiratory function testing with an FEV_1/FVC ratio of less than 0.75.

(4) Asthma†

Acute asthma will not appear in the examination for obvious reasons. A patient in the recovery phase from an acute attack or a patient with the more chronic variety is sometimes included.

Signs
    there may be none
    the patient may be overexpanded or there may be wheeze in the chest
Ask to look at the peak flow chart.

From Fig. 5.1 you ought to note that the patient has morning dips and that there is a gradual increase in the peak flow as the patient recovers. In addition to this there is also a gradual reduction in the diurnal variation in peak flow as the patient recovers. Fig. 5.2 shows a peak flow recorded in chronic asthma. Again note the morning dips around the average of 300 l/min.

You need to know about the assessment and treatment of acute severe asthma (see Chapter 1).

(5) Pleural effusion†

This will usually crop up if there happens to be a patient with a pleural effusion on the ward at the time of the exam. Chronic pleural effusion in out-patients is uncommon.

Signs
    reduced expansion
    stony, dull percussion note

Table 5.2 Signs in respiratory disease. You may find the following table helpful to sort out what is going on inside the chest when you are listening to it.

	Mediastinum	Expansion	Percussion note	Breath sounds	Tactile vocal fremitus
Pleural effusion	Moves away from affected side	→	Stony dull	Absent	→
Pneumothorax	No difference (away from affected side if tension)	→	Hyperresonant	Absent	→
Collapse	Towards affected side	→	→	→ or ← if associated consolidation	→
Consolidation	No change Towards affected if associated collapse	→	→	← or bronchial breathing/ whispering pectoriloquy	←

Note (i) Collapse/consolidation often coexist in real life, and so the signs are mixed.
    (ii) Bronchial breathing and whispering pectoriloquy can be heard above a pleural effusion (sometimes).

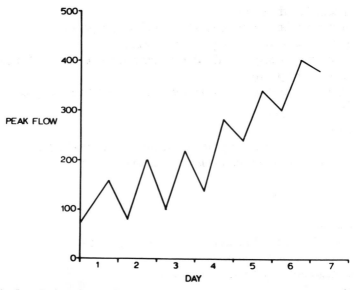

Fig. 5.1   Peak expiratory flow rate of recovery from acute severe asthma. Note the morning 'dipping' improves as the patient recovers.

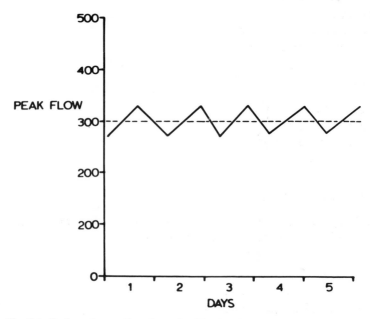

Fig. 5.2   Peak expiratory flow chart of stable chronic asthma.

absent breath sounds
there may be bronchial breathing and/or whispering
pectoriloquy over the top of the effusion
mediastinum may be shifted away from the side of the effusion,
if it is a large one
signs of previous pleural tap, e.g. sticking plaster on patient's
back.

Causes
    (i) think of exudate protein content: greater than 30 g/l.
    (ii) transudate protein content: less than 30 g/l.

Exudate

Neoplastic
    secondary pleural deposits, e.g. from lung or breast*
    primary mesothelioma‡.
Inflammatory — following pneumonia*
    bacterial
    viral
    tubercle.
Pulmonary embolus.
Trauma.
Rheumatoid arthritis, SLE.
Subphrenic abscess, pancreatitis.

Transudate

Heart failure*.
Cirrhosis of liver*.
Nephrotic syndrome‡.
Meig's syndrome‡.

(6) Fibrosing alveolitis†

Although this condition is not that common, the signs are chronic
and such patients are frequently included.

Signs
    clubbing
    central cyanosis
    reduced expansion (bilateral)
    bilateral fine inspiratory crackles worse at bases.

Causes
   idiopathic*
   rheumatoid arthritis
   SLE
   asbestosis.

DRUGS

The idiopathic variety often responds to steroids, so look for the Cushingoid appearance and easy bruising.

Chest X-ray shows reduced lung volumes and fluffy shadows, which start at the bases and work upwards. They make the heart border and diaphragm indistinct.

Respiratory function shows a restrictive deficit with FEV_1/FVC greater than 75% and the vital capacity will invariably be reduced.

(7)   Pneumothorax‡

This is a very rare exam case.

(8)   Sarcoidosis‡

Rare short case. Sometimes included in the long cases.

Signs
   erythema nodosum
   bilateral hilar lymphadenopathy on chest X-ray
   bilateral uveitis
   chest examination is usually normal.

It can also cause (rarely) hepatomegaly, splenomegaly, skin deposits, VII nerve palsies (sometimes bilateral), diffuse CNS involvement. There is often a restrictive defect on the respiratory function tests with an FEV_1/FVC greater than 75% and a reduced transfer factor. If the patient is asymptomatic no treatment is indicated. If the patient is symptomatic, or has widespread disease or worsening transfer factor/X-ray, these patients are treated with prednisolone.

(9)   Haemoptysis

You will occasionally be asked to 'examine this patient who has been coughing up blood'. More commonly you will find blood in the sputum pot (if you remember to look in it) during the course of your examination. Think of the following causes:

Pneumonia (bacterial)*.
Tuberculosis*.
Carcinoma of the lung*.
Bronchiectasis.
Mitral stenosis.
Post-traumatic.
Pulmonary embolus
Idiopathic (this is a common cause in young people in everyday practice, but not in the exam).

(10) Thoracoplasty/physical treatments for TB‡

Patients treated for tuberculosis up until the early 1950s used to have quite drastic surgical procedures as part of their management. They are becoming increasingly scarce as this cohort of patients ages. They are sometimes brought up for the exam.

Thoracoplasty.
Ping pong balls — inserted into upper pleural space to maintain an artificial pneumothorax.

(11) Superior vena cava obstruction‡

This is rare as an examination case, but you need to look for plethora of the upper half of the body and conjunctival suffusion fixed raised JVP, swelling of the arms, face and neck, and collateral vessels. The usual cause is carcinoma of the bronchus impinging on the superior vena cava. It is a 'radiotherapy emergency'. Look for marks on the chest to see if the patient has had or is having a course of radiotherapy.

(12) Cor pulmonale

Students get confused about this. Any chest condition causing prolonged hypoxia will eventually cause pulmonary hypertension. This is due to a direct effect of hypoxia on the pulmonary microcirculation. The pulmonary hypertension, in turn, causes a strain on the right side of the heart. This results in right ventricular hypertrophy and, eventually, right ventricular failure.

Signs
  central cyanosis
  right ventricular heave (felt with the flat of the hand at the left
  sternal edge)
  raised JVP
  peripheral oedema (pitting)
  there may also be hepatomegaly.

You need to remember to look for the causes of the cor pulmonale, e.g. chronic obstructive airways disease or fibrosing
alveolitis.

(13) Pneumonia

Cases of pneumonia in the final MB are uncommon. However, you
may get a patient in the recovery phase.
  You will need to look for signs of consolidation/collapse when
examining the chest. The patient may have residual fever.
  There are many causes of pneumonia but remember the following
headings:

(1) Bacterial, e.g. *Streptococcus pneumoniae*, *Haemophilus
    influenzae*, tuberculosis, *Klebsiella*, *Staphylococcus*.
(2) Viral, including *cytomegalovirus*, *influenza virus*, *RSV*,
    adenovirus, etc.
(3) Rare causes, such as *Pneumocystis carinii*, yeasts and fungi
    (immunocompromised patient).

Mycoplasma can cause pneumonia in otherwise fit adults.

(14) Bronchiectasis

Signs
  clubbing of fingernails
  late inspiratory crackles (often unilateral).

Sputum pot will show purulent, thick secretions and may also
contain blood.
  The pathogenesis involves local dilatation of the bronchi with
subsequent collection of purulent secretions.

Causes
  tuberculosis
  measles

post-nasal drip
foreign body
post-pneumonia
cystic fibrosis
idiopathic.

There is an association with Kartaganer's syndrome. This is a combination of post-nasal drip, bronchiectasis and infertility. This is due to an abnormality of cilial function. Occasionally situs invertus or dextrocardia is found in this syndrome.

KEY QUESTIONS

(1) What are the causes of
   (i) clubbing of the finger nails?
   (ii) pleural effusion?
   (iii) haemoptysis?
   (iv) primary community-acquired chest infections?
   (v) bronchiectasis?
   (vi) cor pulmonale?
(2) How would you differentiate clinically between
   (i) consolidation and collapse?
   (ii) pneumothorax and pleural effusion?
   (iii) peripheral and central cyanosis?
   (iv) restrictive and obstructive airways disease?
(3) Define central cyanosis.

6 The gastrointestinal tract (GIT)

The GIT should be examined in a thorough, systematic way. It is important not to hurt the patient, and before you start your examination you should always ask if the patient has any tenderness in the abdomen. During the course of the examination it is essential to keep glancing at the patient's face, to ensure that you are not causing any discomfort.

The usual question asked in the short case is to either 'examine the GIT' or 'examine the abdomen'. This essentially means a full examination of the GIT, starting at the hands, as set out in Table 6.1. Occasionally you will be asked just to 'palpate the abdomen'. In this case, do exactly what you are told, and no more. However, do not forget to use your eyes, e.g. if you see a fullness in the left hypochondrium make sure you feel particularly thoroughly for a spleen.

The patient should be laid flat in bed. If he is uncomfortable without a pillow, one should be provided. Traditionally the area from knees to nipples should be exposed, but in the exam setting the patient's modesty should be preserved, so the lower limit of exposure should be just above the pubis.

The general scheme for the examination of the GIT is set out in Table 6.1. There are several points to note from this table:

(1) Observation of abdomen

Ask the patient to take a deep breath in whilst observing the abdomen. This accentuates areas of fullness caused by underlying organomegaly/masses.

(2) Palpation

Palpation should be performed from the patient's left side whilst

Table 6.1 Scheme for examination of the GIT

General inspection
Wasting, scars, etc.

Hands
Clubbing (cirrhosis, Crohn's disease.)
Palmar erythema, Dupuytren's contracture, leuconychia (chronic liver disease).

Liver flap
Hepatic encephalopathy.

Conjunctivae
Jaundice, anaemia.

Mouth
Telangiectasia (hereditary haemorrhagic telangiectasia)
Perioral pigmentation (Peutz-Jegher syndrome).

Tongue

Supraclaviclar nodes
Virchow's node, Troisier's sign.

Skin on chest wall
Spider naevi, gynaecomastia, bruising/purpura (chronic liver disease).

Observation of abdomen
Areas of fullness
  masses
  organomegaly
  ascites.
Scars (see Fig. 6.1)
Distended veins on the anterior abdominal wall. Determine direction of blood flow (see Fig. 6.2.)
Everted umbilicus (ascites; several litres of fluid needed to produce this sign).
Visible peristalsis (bowel obstruction).

Palpation
Light and deep, do each quadrant in turn.
Feel for masses, organomegaly (liver, kidneys, spleen, bladder, uterus) and tenderness. Remember to look at the patient's face.

Percussion
Areas of dullness corresponding to masses/organomegaly.

Shifting dullness/fluid thrill (see Plates 1 + 2)

Auscultation
Bowel sounds — bruits (renal artery, aortic, hepatic).
'Liver scratch sign' (Fig. 6.3).
Extra thinking time (see Chapter 1).
Hernial orifices.
Peripheral oedema (hypoalbuminaemia).
Do not examine genitals or do a PR unless examiner asks. Ask if this required.

kneeling or sitting. The reason for this is that the hand is more relaxed, and more in contact with the patient in this position. It is far more sensitive than examining the patient whilst you are in the standing position.

Liver

Start in the right iliac fossa (RIF) and work upwards, asking the patient to breathe in as you palpate.

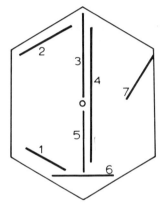

Fig. 6.1 Abdominal scars.
1 Appendix. 2 Cholecystectomy. 3 Gastric surgery. 4 Laparotomy.
5 Hysterectomy/Classical Caesarian. 6 Caesarian section. 7 Nephrectomy.

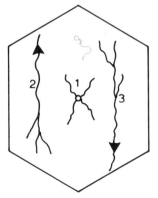

Fig. 6.2 Abnormal anterior abdominal veins. 1 *Caput medusae*. Dilated veins around the umbilicus, found in portal hypertension: flow is away from the umbilicus. 2 *IVC obstruction*: flow upwards. 3 *SVC obstruction*: flow downwards.

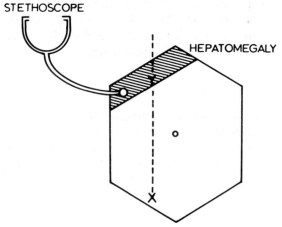

Fig. 6.3 The liver scratch sign. This technique is helpful to confirm the presence of hepatomegaly, suspected by palpation and percussion. It is particularly useful in the obese patient, when percussion and palpation of organs may be difficult. Listen with the stethoscope over the liver edge. At the same time lightly scratch the abdominal wall with the fingernail in the right iliac fossa (point X). Work your way upwards, scratching gently as you go. When you come over the liver edge (point Y), you will hear a loud scratching noise. This is because the scratching sound is being transmitted through the liver substance, which is solid and therefore a good sound conductor.

Spleen

Start in the RIF and work towards the left hypochondrium. If you start in the left iliac fossa (LIF) or left hypochondrium you may miss a very large spleen.

To feel a small spleen it may be necessary to get the patient to roll partly on to the right side and feel with the fingertips under the left costal margin (during inspiration).

(3) Percussion

Percuss the whole abdomen. Remember to percuss the upper border of the liver and spleen.

(4) Ascites

Shifting dullness

Percuss out the anterior limit of the fluid level. This is best done with your finger parallel to the air/fluid interface (i.e. in the sagittal plane — see Plate 1). Now ask the patient to roll on to their side. Repercuss to assess if the area of dullness has moved, which indicates free fluid in the peritoneal space.

Fluid thrill

If you have demonstrated shifting dullness, go on to try to demonstrate a fluid thrill. Ask the examiner to firmly place the hypothenar aspect of his hand on the midline of the anterior abdominal wall (in the sagittal plane). Flick the fluid at one side, whilst palpating the other (see Plate 2).

TYPICAL CASES

(1) Hepatomegaly*

Delineate the lower border of the liver, and size it in terms of finger breadths below the costal margin. Remember also to find where the upper border is (by percussion). This is important because occasionally a liver edge can be felt just below the costal margin when there is no true hepatomegaly, e.g. chronic obstructive airways disease where hyperexpanded lungs push down the (normal-sized) liver.

Define the characteristics of the liver edge you have felt in terms of:
  (i) The edge
        smooth
        knobbly (multiple metastases).
 (ii) Pulsatility (tricuspid regurgitation).
(iii) Consistency
        firm
        hard.
 (iv) Bruit (hepatocellular carcinoma, a-v malformation).
  (v) Tenderness (hepatitis, capsular pain of the hepatomegaly of congestive cardiac failure).

Think of the causes of hepatomegaly and look for other signs which may give you the diagnosis of the patient in front of you (see Table 6.2).

Table 6.2   Hepatomegaly: causes and signs to look for

Cause	Signs to look for
Cirrhosis*	Chronic liver disease
Fatty infiltration*	Alcohol abuse (may be no other signs)
Congestive cardiac failure (CCF)*	JVP Signs of LVF 　crackles at the bases 　third heart sound
Metastatic carcinoma†	Look for the site of primary 　breasts 　lung 　prostate, etc.
Hepatitis‡ (A, B, C)	Jaundice, splenomegaly, tattoos, signs of i.v. drug abuse Ask about travel, transfusions, sexual history
Hepatoma‡	Listen for bruit Ask about past history of hepatitis B/cirrhosis
Lymphoma‡	Splenomegaly, lymphadenopathy, fever, weight loss
Leukaemia (all types)‡	Splenomegaly, nodes (CLL), purpura, petechiae, fever, etc.

Notes:

(1) In the later stages of cirrhosis the liver is impalpable, as it is small, shrunken and fibrosed.
(2) Very rare exam cases:
　Sarcoid.
　TB.
　Infectious mononucleosis (EB virus, CMV, toxoplasmosis).

(2) Splenomegaly*

A favourite examiners' question is 'how can you tell the difference clinically between splenomegaly and a palpable left kidney?'

Answer

Spleen has a notch, kidney does not.
You can ballot a kidney, you cannot ballot a spleen.

Can't get above spleen

---

* Very common.
† Common.
‡ Rare and/or difficult.

Percussion
kidney resonant (unreliable)
spleen dull.
You cannot get above a spleen, you sometimes can get above a kidney. (I never have, except a transplanted or horse-shoe kidney.)

Splenomegaly is subjectively categorised as mild, moderate or large.

Large (past umbilicus)
chronic granulocytic leukaemia
myelofibrosis
kala-azar[‡] (*not* in UK).
Moderate (up to the umbilicus)[†]
lymphoma
chronic lymphatic leukaemia (CLL)
portal hypertension
malaria[‡].
Mild (just palpable)[†]
portal hypertension
lymphoma
CLL
polycythaemia rubra vera
rheumatoid arthritis (ask to see full blood count result — Felty's syndrome)
SLE[‡]
amyloidosis
hepatitis
infectious mononucleosis   } Rare in the exam
malaria.

(3) Hepatosplenomegaly★

Causes
cirrhosis and portal hypertension★
chronic right-sided heart failure[†]
lymphoma
leukaemia (any type)
infections[‡]
    hepatitis (A, B, C)
    infectious mononucleosis, TB
amyloid[‡]
sarcoid[‡].

(4) Chronic liver disease★

Very common case. Think of the signs. Look for signs of complications. Think about the causes.

Signs
  palmar erythema★
  spider naevi★
  gynaecomastia[†]
  testicular atrophy[†]
  hepatomegaly[†]
  ascites[†]
  peripheral oedema[†]
  jaundice[†]
  muscle wasting[†]
  clubbing of the fingernails[‡]
  central cyanosis[‡] ('intrapulmonary spider naevi' causing shunting)
  liver flap   ⎫
  hepatic fetor   ⎬ Hepatic encephalopathy
  inability to draw five-pointed star   ⎪
  mental obtundation.   ⎭
Complications
  portal hypertension
    splenomegaly,
    abnormal abdominal veins (see Fig. 6.2),
    oesophageal varices (bleeding)
  gram-negative sepsis
  hepatoma (in cirrhosis).
Causes
  alcoholic cirrhosis★
  idiopathic cirrhosis★
  chronic active hepatitis[†]
  chronic hepatitis B infection[†]
  rare — drugs, e.g. methyldopa, isoniazid
  primary biliary cirrhosis
  haemachromatosis
  Wilson's disease.

(5) Ascites [†]

You need to examine for this in the correct manner, as described earlier in the chapter. Fullness in both flanks on general inspection usually gives the game away (the only other common cause for this is polycystic disease of the kidneys). Look for an everted umbilicus.

Causes

The commonest cause, by far, is cirrhosis of the liver. It is helpful to think of the causes under the following headings:

hypoalbuminaemia
    cirrhosis*
    protein — calorie malnutrition
    nephrotic syndrome
    protein-losing enteropathy.
portal hypertension — cirrhosis*
local inflammatory process
    metastatic carcinoma (in the peritoneum)
    pelvic carcinoma (ovary)
    infection (e.g. peritoneal TB).

Note: Constrictive pericarditis causes ascites (and gross hepato-megaly), whilst causing very little peripheral oedema.

(6) Portal hypertension (see earlier)

Causes
    cirrhosis*
    portal vein occlusion — carcinoma of head of pancreas, portal
                       vein thrombosis
    Budd–Chiari syndrome‡ (occlusion of hepatic veins).

(7) Jaundice

The patient will almost invariably be an in-patient. This fact makes jaundice an uncommon examination case. You are more likely to meet jaundice as a long case.
    Remember the basic causes:

Pre-hepatic
    autoimmune haemolytic anaemia
    drug-induced haemolytic anaemia (e.g. methyldopa)
    hereditary spherocytosis
    sickle cell anaemia
    thalassaemias

transfusion reactions[‡]
red cell fragmentation syndromes[‡]
(e.g. DIC secondary to septicaemia)
Gilbert's syndrome[†]
Hepatic[†]
   cirrhosis (any cause)
   alcoholic liver disease*
   chronic active hepatitis
   hepatitis (A, B, non-A non-B, glandular fever, Weil's disease)[‡]
   metastatic carcinoma of the liver
   hepatotoxic drugs (e.g. post-paracetamol overdose, halothane).
Cholestasis
   drugs, e.g. chlorpromazine
   biliary obstruction
      gallstones
      carcinoma of pancreas
      cholangitis.

History

The patients will complain of jaundice, itching, dark urine and pale stools (cholestasis). Points to look out for are:

Transfusions.
Travel.
Tattoos.   } Hepatitis
Drug abuse (intravenous).
Sexual preferences.
Infectious contacts.
Job (sewers) — Weil's disease[‡]
Family history of jaundice or splenectomy (suggests haemolysis).
Past history of recurrent jaundice
   haemolysis
   Gilbert's syndrome.
Drug history (see above).
Alcohol intake.
Back/abdominal pains (pancreatitis/carcinoma of pancreas).
Ulcerative colitis/fever/jaundice — cholangitis.

Examination

Look for:

Stigmata of chronic liver disease.

Hepatomegaly (knobbly in secondary carcinoma).
Splenomegaly (haemolysis or portal hypertension).
Anaemia (haemolysis).
Palpable gallbladder (carcinoma of pancreas).
Needle puncture marks (hepatitis B).

Patients with haemolytic jaundice have a lemon yellow tinge.

Investigation

Raised unconjugated bilirubin.
Urobilinogen in urine.   Imply haemolytic
Reduced haptoglobins.   jaundice

Remember the Coombe's test, Hb electrophoresis and red cell fragility studies.

The ALT and AST are raised out of proportion to the alkaline phosphatase in hepatic jaundice.

Alkaline phosphatase is raised out of proportion to ALT in cholestasis. Ultrasound examination is essential to determine the calibre of the common bile duct. If this is dilated it implies a surgical (cholestatic) cause for the jaundice.

(8) Malabsorption[‡]

This is an uncommon case in finals. You are only likely to meet it in the long case section.

(9) Anaemia

You will usually meet this as a long case.

Hypochromic microcytic

Iron deficiency due to:

Chronic blood loss
   peptic ulcer
   carcinoma of the stomach, colon or caecum
   colitis
   uterine
   renal tract[‡].

Malabsorption secondary to partial gastrectomy, extensive ileal resection, coeliac disease.
Dietary.
During pregnancy.

Normochromic normocytic

Chronic disease
   rheumatoid arthritis
   systemic lupus erythematosus
   Crohn's disease
   carcinoma
   lymphoma
   chronic infections, e.g. TB.

Macrocytic

B12 deficiency (this can be due to dietary causes, although this is rare, e.g. in veganism).
More common causes are secondary to malabsorption
   pernicious anaemia
   gastrectomy
   blind-loop syndrome
   tropical sprue
   ileal resection
   Crohn's disease.
Folate deficiency
   dietary (alcoholics, old age, pregnancy)
   malabsorption (see above)
   increased utilisation of folate (pregnancy, haemolysis, myelosclerosis, carcinoma)
   anticonvulsant therapy.

KEY QUESTIONS

(1) What are the causes of
    (i) ascites?
    (ii) hepatomegaly?
    (iii) splenomegaly?
    (iv) hepatosplenomegaly?
    (v) liver bruit?
    (vi) cirrhosis?
    (vii) jaundice?
    (viii) diarrhoea?
    (ix) constipation?
    (x) anaemia
        hypochromic microcytic?
        normochromic normocytic?
        megaloblastic?
    (xi) macrocytosis (without anaemia)?

(2) What are the signs of chronic liver disease?

(3) What is the difference clinically between splenomegaly and an enlarged left kidney?

7 Renal medicine

Renal medicine is regarded by some as a postgraduate subject. Having said this, on occasion you will meet a renal patient in finals. However, there are only a very limited selection of cases that you are likely to encounter. The likelihood of coming across renal cases in finals varies up and down the country. It essentially depends on your teaching hospital's access to renal patients, dialysis centres, etc. Ask colleagues about what has happened in previous years, as the pattern is likely to repeat itself.

You need to know how to examine the kidneys, and how to distinguish between an enlarged left kidney and an enlarged spleen (see Chapter 6).

TYPICAL CASES

(1) Polycystic kidneys*

This is the commonest renal case in finals.

Clinical features
bilaterally palpable kidneys, which feel lobulated (multiple cysts)
hypertension
signs of chronic renal failure (see later)
examine urine for blood/protein/casts
ask about the family history

Polycystic disease of the kidneys is an autosomal dominant condition. There are multiple cysts in the kidneys (and sometimes liver). Patients develop chronic renal failure during adult life and are usually on some form of renal support (dialysis/transplant) by their 40s.

Complications
hypertension

recurrent urinary tract infections
haemorrhage into a cyst
ruptured Berry aneurysm (Berry aneurysms are more common in polycystic disease).

(2) Bilateral renal enlargement

Causes
    polycystic kidneys*
    bilateral hydronephrosis[†]
    amyloidosis[‡].

(3) Unilateral enlarged kidney

Causes
    hydronephrosis
    renal carcinoma
    simple renal cysts (benign)
    hypertrophy of single kidney
    transplanted kidney (left iliac fossa, usually).

(4) Chronic renal failure

You are more likely to meet this as a long case. It is sometimes seen as a short case.

Symptoms
    malaise
    tiredness
    bone pain (osteomalacia) etc.
Signs
    brown line on fingernails
    yellow colouration to skin
    anaemia (reduced erythropoietin production)
    hypertension
    signs of fluid overload (raised JVP, peripheral oedema).

---

* Very common.
[†] Common.
[‡] Rare and/or difficult.

Signs of renal support
  fistula   ⎫
  shunt   ⎬ haemodialysis
  peritoneal dialysis
  renal transplant.

You need to look for signs which may tell you the cause of the patient's chronic renal failure.

Causes
  glomerulonephritis*
  pyelonephritis[†]
  diabetes[†]
  hypertension[†]
  polycystic disease of the kidneys[†].

8 Endocrinology

Endocrinology cases are straightforward, so long as you have prepared yourself properly for them.

You will appreciate that there is no particular organ system to examine: your examination should be tailored to the patient in front of you, and may involve examining parts of several 'systems'.

TYPICAL CASES

(1) The diabetic★

It would be unusual for you not to come across a diabetic patient at some stage in the exam. Diabetics are either insulin (IDDM) or non-insulin dependent (NIDDM).

Ask about *symptoms*:

Presenting
  weight loss, polyuria, polydipsia, dizziness, blurred vision, etc.
Of complications
  e.g. pins and needles (peripheral neuropathy)
  visual problems (? new vessel formation)
  leg ulcers (infected feet)
  vomiting ⎫
  nocturnal diarrhoea ⎬ autonomic neuropathy
  impotence ⎭
  postural hypotension
  intermittent claudication (peripheral vascular disease).

Signs

You are looking for the signs of the complications of diabetes.

Skin
Necrobiosis lipoidica (yellow lesions on the shins, usually).

Leg ulcers.
Infected feet/toes.
Injection sites (sometimes get fat atrophy which leaves skin hollowed out).
Xanthelasmata (associated hyperlipidaemia).
granuloma annulare.

CVS

Absent pulses in the lower limbs (peripheral vascular disease).
Retinal changes
    haemorrhages
    exudates
    new vessels
    laser treatment.
Autonomic neuropathy (postural hypotension). (This is confirmed by ECGs taken before, during and after a Valsalva manoeuvre and looking for changes in the R–R interval).

CNS

Sensory ('glove and stocking') neuropathy.
Diabetic amyotrophy (femoral nerve damage causing wasting of quadriceps and absent knee jerk).
Mononeuritis multiplex (multiple peripheral nerve palsies).
Charcot's joints — painless, disorganised joint in a patient with a peripheral neuropathy.

Urogenital system. Signs of chronic renal failure (see Chapter 7).

Make sure you ask to examine the urine. You will be looking for:

(1) Glucose:
    ? compliance with treatment
    ? correct level of treatment
    Ask to look at a series of urine glucoses (or BM Stix).
(2) protein: microscopic albuminuria is the first sign of diabetic renal disease, and should be carefully screened for.
(3) ketones.

You need to know about the treatment and follow-up of diabetics. Spend a couple of sessions in the diabetic clinic if you have never been.

You will be asked about the new monocomponent insulins. You need to know how these differ from the older varieties.

The 'assessment and management of diabetic ketoacidosis' is a common written question and is not infrequently asked in the viva. Look these topics up in a standard text.

Causes of diabetes

Idiopathic (95%).
Steroid therapy[†], thiazide diuretics.
Pancreatitis, post-pancreatectomy.
Haemochromatosis.
Cushing's syndrome.
Acromegaly, phaeochromocytoma.

(2) Hyperthyroidism

This is not a common case: most patients will be on, or have had, some form of treatment and will therefore (hopefully) be euthyroid.
  The diagnosis is usually given away by the typical facial appearance, with bulging eyes. However, the specific signs to look for are:

Agitation, sweating.
Tremor (exaggerated physiological tremor).
Resting tachycardia.
Atrial fibrillation.
Exophthalmos.
Lid lag/lid retraction.
Goitre.
Bruit over the thyroid.
Pretibial myxoedema[‡].

  Rarely thyrotoxicosis may cause a proximal myopathy.

(3) Goitre

You may be asked to 'examine this patient's goitre'.
  Follow the simple scheme of:

Look.
Feel.
Percuss (retrosternal goitre).
Listen.

Look at the contours of the patient's neck from the front and the side. If it is a goitre there will be a swelling between the thyroid cartilage and the manubrium sternum. It may be mainly unilateral, particularly if there is a single nodule in the thyroid.

Now go behind the patient to palpate the thyroid with the flat of both hands (best done with the patient sitting in a chair). Ask the patient to have a sip from a glass of water and hold the water in her mouth. When you are ready ask her to swallow whilst palpating the thyroid. If the swelling goes up on swallowing, the diagnosis is that of a goitre.

Now assess the characteristics of the goitre:

Smooth
    Graves' disease
    simple goitre (iodine-deficient)
    multiple cysts
    multinodular goitre.
Single nodule
    carcinoma of the thyroid
    benign adenoma
    single simple cyst.
Tender
    thyroiditis.

If you feel a single nodule, feel for local lymph nodes and attachment to local structures in the neck. These are features of malignant thyroid nodule. Remember to listen for a bruit over the thyroid (ask the patient to hold her breath). This is sometimes heard in Graves' disease with a very vascular thyroid.

You must now look for signs of hyper-or hypothyroidism (see 2 and 4).

(4) Hypothyroidism[†]

Again this is not a common examination case, for reasons given above.

Causes
    idiopathic atrophy*
    post-^{131}I therapy*
    post-thyroidectomy*
    post-Hashimoto's thyroiditis[‡]

Signs
   psychomotor retardation
   dry scaly skin
   'peaches and cream' complexion
   dry brittle hair, hair loss
   loss of outer third of eyebrow (unreliable sign)
   goitre
   hoarse voice
   weight gain
   sinus bradycardia
   carpal tunnel syndrome
   slow-relaxing reflexes
   cardiomyopathy[‡]
   dementia[‡]
   peripheral neuropathy[‡]
   cerebellar degeneration[‡].

(5) Acromegaly[†]

This is caused by a growth hormone-secreting adenoma in the pituitary gland. Even after treatment with bromocriptine or hypophysectomy (or both) the patient will still have residual signs of his disease. So, although acromegaly is a rare condition in everyday clinical practice, it is relatively common in the examination setting.

Signs
   prominent jaw
                nose
                orbital ridges
   large hands
   large feet
   typical facies
   large, burly stature.

Remember to examine the visual fields for bitemporal hemianopia, which is caused by a local pressure effect of the tumour on the optic chiasm.

Complications of acromegaly
   hypertension
   proximal myopathy
   carpal tunnel syndrome
   osteoarthrosis (particularly of lower limbs)

cardiomyopathy (this is not infrequently the cause of death in the patient's 50s or 60s).
Associated conditions
diabetes
hypopituitarism
hypercalcaemia.

(6) Cushing's syndrome

This syndrome is due to excess circulating corticosteroids.

Causes
  (i) iatrogenic* — patients with conditions such as asthma or systemic lupus erythematosis are not infrequently treated with oral steroids and may exhibit some of the signs of Cushing's syndrome
 (ii) Cushing's disease‡ — ACTH-secreting pituitary adenoma adrenal cortical adenoma‡
(iii) ectopic ACTH from bronchial carcinoma.
       The commonest cause, by far, is the iatrogenic variety.

Signs
    moon face
    fragile skin
    easy bruising
    buffalo hump
    striae (abdominal wall)
    hirsuitism
    muscular wasting
    proximal myopathy.

Patients with Cushing's syndrome are more likely to develop diabetes, hypertension, recurrent infections and bone fractures (osteoporotic).

Note. Nelson's syndrome occurs after adrenalectomy for Cushing's disease. The main features are of pigmentation associated with the increase in circulating ACTH which follows such an operation.

(7) Addison's disease‡

In this condition there are insufficient circulating corticosteroids due to failure of the adrenal cortex.

Causes
 idiopathic* (autoimmune and associated with diabetes and thyroid disease)
 metastatic deposits in the adrenal cortex from a primary in the lung or breast
 tuberculosis‡ (calcified adrenals on plain abdominal X-ray)
Symptoms
 weight loss
 lassitude
 postural hypotension
 visual disturbance
 vomiting
Signs
 pigmentation
  hand (palmar creases)
  knee
  buccal
  generalised
 postural hypotension
 fluid depletion.

The urea and electrolytes show hyponatraemia and hyper-kalaemia.

(8) Hypopituitarism‡

Rare case.

(9) Phaeochromocytoma‡

Very rare exam case.

KEY QUESTIONS

(1) What are the causes of
   (i) diabetes?
   (ii) goitre?
   (iii) Cushing's syndrome?
   (iv) Addison's disease?
(2) What clinical features suggest a malignant goitre?
(3) Describe the more unusual ways in which the following diseases may present
   (i) diabetes.
   (ii) thyrotoxicosis.
   (iii) hypothyroidism.
   (iv) Addison's disease.
   (v) Cushing's disease.
(4) What abnormalities are found in the serum glucose and urea and electrolytes in
   (i) Addison's disease?
   (ii) Cushing's disease?

9 Dermatology

N. J. Reynolds MB BS BSc MRCP

Skin disease is very common but is not examined in detail in the MB exam. Candidates are presented either with common dermatological conditions or important dermatological manifestations of systemic disease.

Scheme for history of skin conditions

Initial lesion(s)
Site.
Duration.
Spread.
Exacerbating/relieving factors.

PMH
Associated conditions.

Drugs
Dermatological side effects are very common.
May exacerbate pre-existing skin disease.

SH
Environmental factors — work environment, travel abroad, sun exposure.
The impact of the skin condition on the patient's life must be assessed.

FH
Many skin conditions have an hereditary component.

Scheme for examination of the skin

Examine the whole skin surface including nails, mouth, eyes and scalp in a long case.
Ensure optimal lighting — bedside lighting is often inadequate.
Look and then palpate.
Assess
  single or multiple lesions★
  colour
  surface change — ? scaling
  margin — ill or well-defined
  temperature
  depth of lesion
  distribution.

TYPICAL CASES

If presented with a dermatological long case I would recommend an initial brief examination of the skin as the diagnosis may then be apparent allowing a more appropriate and relevant history to be taken.

(1) Psoriasis

Very common.

Look for
    well-defined scaly plaques
    guttate lesions
    pustules (especially hands and feet)
    evidence of the Koebner phenomenon
    nail changes (pitting and onycholysis)
    scalp involvement
    arthropathy.

★Descriptive terms
Macule   —   flat lesion.
Papule   —   circumscribed raised lesion <1 cm diameter.
Nodule   —   circumscribed raised lesion >1 cm diameter.
Vesicle, bulla —   fluid-filled lesion.
Pustule   —   pus-filled lesion.

Ask about
   exacerbating factors
      sore throats (streptococcal infection)
      life events and stress
      skin trauma including sunburn
   FH
   previous therapy.

(2) Dermatitis

May be due to:

(a) Atopic eczema

Common.

Onset often in early childhood.
Widespread, symmetrical ill-defined areas of itchy red
papulovesicles involving particularly the flexural aspects
of elbows and knees. Lichenification may be prominent.
Ask about
   PH or FH of atopy
   exacerbating factors
   details of therapy.

(b) Contact Dermatitis

Uncommon.

Consider when 'eczema' is localised, asymmetrical or of late onset.
Ask about
   occupation
   hobbies
   topical medicaments.

Recommend patch testing.

(c) Seborrhoeic Dermatitis

Rare, but common in HIV disease.

(d) Varicose Eczema

(3) **Lichen planus**

Rare

Grouped, very itchy, violaceous flat-topped papules.
Look for
    nail changes — pterygium formation
    mucosal change — Wickham's striae
    Koebner phenomenon.

(4) **Bullous Disorders**

Rare.

Pemphigoid

Subepidermal tense, intact blisters.
Age onset 65–75 years.
Mucous membrane involvement uncommon.

Pemphigus Vulgaris

Intraepidermal flaccid or deroofed blisters.
Age onset 40–60 years.
Mucous membrane involvement very common.

Dermatitis Herpetiformis

Small, very itchy subepidermal blisters on extensor surfaces —
often excoriated.
Age onset 20–55 years.
Associated with gluten-sensitive enteropathy.

Other Causes

Congenital (epidermolysis bullosa).
Trauma.
Insect bite reaction.
Infections (staphylococcal scalded skin syndrome).
Photosensitivity.
Drugs (barbiturates).
Erythema multiforme.

(5) Erythema Nodosum

Common.

Causes
  infections
    streptococcal
    TB
  sarcoidosis
  inflammatory bowel disease
  drugs (sulphonamides).

(6) Generalised hyperpigmentation

Uncommon.

Causes
  Addison's disease
  malabsorption
  haemochromatosis
  drugs (chlorpromazine).

(7) Leg Ulceration

Very common.

Causes
  venous
  arterial
  diabetic
  malignant
  pyoderma gangrenosum
  sickle cell disease
  vasculitis.
Ask about
  intermittent claudication
  PH of DVT.
Assess
  arterial system — peripheral pulses
  venous system — varicose veins
  skin — varicose eczema.

Necrobiosis lipoidica and pretibial myxoedema will be covered in Chapter 12.

(8) Malignant Melanoma

Uncommon but may come up in the viva.
Distinguishing clinical features from a benign pigmented lesion are:

Absolute size (benign moles usually < 1 cm diameter).
Increasing size.
Irregular outline.
Irregular pigment distribution.
Changing colour.
Itching.
Bleeding.
Ulceration.
Raised nodules.

KEY QUESTIONS

(1) With which condition is dermatitis herpetiformis associated?
(2) What internal disorders may produce generalised pruritus?
(3) How may contact dermatitis be distinguished from atopic dermatitis?
(4) What are the cutaneous manifestations of internal malignancy?

10 Neurology

Neurological cases are regarded with some trepidation by many candidates. There are several reasons for this. Neurological disease can result in many signs, some of which carry rather long and unpronounceable names. A good neurological examination is an art form: when performed by an expert it can be a pleasure to watch. This is rarely the case in the examination room.

Candidates are sometimes wrong-footed by the question 'where is the lesion?'. Unfortunately, to give a meaningful answer you need to understand basic neuroanatomy: this raises the spectre of the dreaded (but long-forgotten) second MB.

Before you start this chapter I recommend you acquaint yourself with the following information from a standard anatomy textbook

(1) Sensory pathways.
(2) Motor pathways.
(3) Sensory dermatomes.
(4) Root values of
    peripheral nerves
    muscle groups
    reflex arcs.
(5) Gross anatomy of the brain, including brain stem, cranial nerves and their nuclei.

The most important thing to remember about a neurological examination is that it is *comparative*. In other words you test one sign on one side and then test on the other and compare the difference. Do not forget to do this at all times: the examiners will be looking closely for it.

In the examination room you will never be asked to do a full neurological examination in the short cases: this would take far too long. Instead, the examiner will ask you to examine part of the nervous system (e.g. arms, legs, cranial nerves, cerebellum, etc.).

Table 10.1

	UMN	LMN
Observation	—	Wasting, fasciculation
Tone	Spasticity	Hypotonicity
Power	Weakness	Weakness
Reflexes	Hyper-reflexia Extensor plantars Clonus	Hyporeflexia

You must be practised at doing such bits of a full neurological examination. It is for this reason that this chapter has been divided into the sections of 'regional neurology' as set out below:

(1) The head
     eyes
     cranial nerves
     speech
     higher functions.
(2) Upper limb.
(3) Lower limb.
(4) Abnormal gait and movements.
(5) Diffuse disease.

Many neurological problems will extend beyond the region you have been asked to examine. You must appreciate this and be seen to appreciate it by the examiners. For example if you find ataxic nystagmus when asked to examine the eyes, you must be seen to look for other signs of multiple sclerosis.

Before you start the rest of the chapter it is important to appreciate the difference between upper motor neurone (UMN) and lower motor neurone (LMN) lesions (frequently) asked question — see Table 10.1).

Try to look stylish when you swing the patella hammer.

(1) THE HEAD

(a) EYES

Examination of the eyes causes mortal fear in some candidates. Actually this is unnecessary: eye cases are usually rather simple.

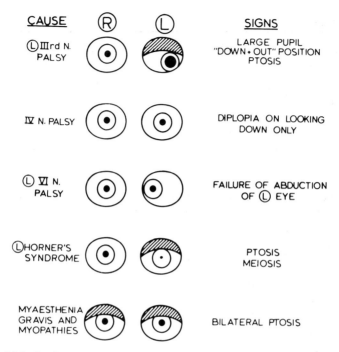

Fig. 10.1 Pupillary and eyelid abnormalities.

You need to have a good scheme for examination, a grasp of the essentials of using an ophthalmoscope and a knowledge of the cases which you are likely to meet.

Scheme for the examination of the eyes

Observation
Look at the patient's eyes at rest. The diagnosis may be obvious, e.g. exophthalmos (thyrotoxicosis), Horner's syndrome, etc. (see Fig. 10.1).

Also look for xanthelasmata, senile arcus, etc.

Feel
Feel for increased tone in the eyes (palpation). This is a very inaccurate way of assessing intraocular pressure, which is normally measured by a very sensitive machine. Intraocular pressure is raised in conditions such as glaucoma.

Visual acuity

Test this by asking the patient to read some small print (with glasses if he wears them), e.g. from a newspaper. A more formal assessment can be made with standard Snellen charts.

Visual fields

Sit on the edge of the patient's bed. Equilibrate the patient's visual fields with your own by making sure your heads are at the same level, 1 m apart. Ask the patient to cover one eye. Now cover your own eye (the opposite one to the one patient has just covered). Test the patient's visual field (against your own) by slowly bringing a finger or white hat-pin from outside your field of vision (whilst the patient looks into your uncovered eye). Bring the hat-pin in at 2, 4, 8 and 10 o'clock, as this will pick up quadrantic field defects better.

Now, using a red hat-pin, assess the blind spot (against your own) and look for scotomata (see common field defect, Fig. 10.2).

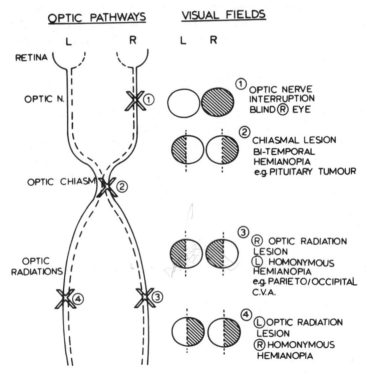

Fig. 10.2 Visual fields defects.

Fundoscopy

It is essential to be familiar with the ophthalmoscope you use during the examination. The only way to ensure that this happens is by taking either your own or one which you have borrowed. The patient should be in a darkened room with dilated pupils (ask for mydriatic drops if necessary).

Set the machine with a plain lens and normal filters. Shine it onto your hand to check it is working. Now elicit the red reflex in both of the patient's eyes. This is done by shining the light through the pupil from about 0.5 m. Light hits the retina and is reflected back as a red glow as you look through the lens of the ophthalmascope. Anything which causes an interruption to this pathway of light will cause an absent red reflex, e.g:

Cataract.
Prosthetic eye.
Haemorrhage into anterior chamber.
Vitreous haemorrhage.

Now examine the eye itself. Start off by asking the patient to look at a spot in the distance, ignoring the light of the ophthalmoscope. Approach the patient's eye from a slightly lateral direction. This approach has two advantages:

(1) It enables the patient to concentrate on the spot in the distance, with minimal disturbance to his field of vision.
(2) The optic disc should pop straight into view. (Focus on the optic disc by altering the lens strength to get a sharp image.) For short-sighted patients you will need a negative lens and for long-sighted patients you will need a positive lens. Once you have found the disc your problems should be over. Examine it carefully and assess:

Colour.
Margin.
Contour.

If you cannot find the disc follow the vessels until it comes into view.
Look at all areas of the retina and in particular:

Vessels
    tortuosity
    silver wiring
    a-v nipping

    new vessel formation
    haemorrhages.
Retinal surface
    haemorrhages
    exudates
    evidence of laser therapy.

Now slowly 'rack back' by increasing the lens strength of the ophthalmoscope. Check the posterior chamber, lens (for cataracts) and anterior chamber.

With practice fundoscopy will become easier. Examine as many normal fundi as possible. Remember that negroid and Asian retinae look much darker than caucasian ones.

Move

You will be essentially testing cranial nerves III, IV and VI and the intraocular muscles which they supply.

Stand to the left of the patient. Rest your left hand on the patient's forehead (to help keep it still) . Now, asking the patient to follow the index finger of your right hand, test all directions of movement. Ask the patient to say 'yes' if he sees double. Try to find out in which direction of gaze the double vision is worst.

Look for
    failure of gaze (and direction)
    nystagmus
    dysconjugate gaze.

Note: Make sure you do not confuse physiological and pathological nystagmus. To avoid this mistake remember the following two tips:

Do not draw the patient's gaze too far laterally.
Do not place the finger too close to the patient's eyes (0.5 m is usually ideal).

A colleague of mine never quite mastered the art of fundoscopy. This seems to have started on the French skiing slopes, which is where he was to be found during the majority of his ophthalmology attachment. When it came to the assessment at the end of the term he felt rather vulnerable. Being an enterprising sort, he wandered up to the ophthalmology ward the day before and learnt by heart all the patients' names and relevant diagnoses. The day of the test arrived and he was called into the examination room. The consultant introduced the patient — a Mr Ferguson. A wave of confidence swept through the candidate. He looked thoughtfully at the patient's eyes (from a distance), stroked his chin in consideration and then, without so much as touching the ophthalmoscope said:

'I think it is a case of optic atrophy, Sir!'

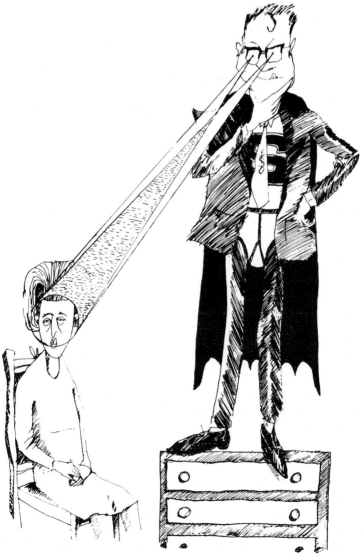

'Hmm . . . . , another case of optic atrophy.'

TYPICAL CASES

(1) **Fundoscopy**

Diabetes★ (see Plate 3)

Look for
  haemorrhages
  exudates
  new vessel formation
  signs of laser therapy

Cataracts are more common in diabetics.

Hypertension

Look for
  vessel tortuosity (unreliable sign)
  silver-wiring
  a-v nipping
  haemorrhages
  papilloedema.

Papilloedema is only present in cases of malignant hypertension, which is extremely rare.

Optic atrophy

If the disc looks surprisingly white, distinct and much easier to find than normal, it is probably optic atrophy. It is absolutely essential to compare it with the disc on the other side (see Plate 4).

Causes
  multiple sclerosis
  post-traumatic
  retro-orbital tumour
  diabetes
  retinal artery thrombosis.

Cochosu !!

★ Very common.
† Common.
‡ Rare and/or difficult.

Papilloedema

The disc edges are blurred and impossible to focus properly by adjusting the lenses of the ophthalmoscope. The disc itself may also be blurred and pink. Look for exudates and haemorrhages. Compare with the other side (see Plate 5).

Hint: If you find the disc difficult or impossible to find, papilloedema is probably present.

Causes
    raised intracranial pressure, e.g. tumour
    abscess
    benign intracranial hypertension[‡]
    malignant hypertension[‡].

Glass eye

Some nasty examiners will ask you to do fundoscopy on a prosthetic eye. If you remember to do the red reflex first you will stay one step ahead.

(2) Ptosis (drooping of the eyelid)

Causes
    third nerve palsy (large pupil)
    part of Horner's syndrome (small pupil)
    myopathies (usually bilateral ptosis)
        myaesthenia gravis
        myotonia congenita
        other congenital myopathies, e.g. facio/scapulo humeral
    idiopathic.

Note: Bilateral ptosis, particularly if mild, can be difficult to spot.

(3) Horner's syndrome

This is rare in practice, but common in exams. There is a classical combination of signs, which is:

Ptosis.
Enophthalmos.
Meiosis (small pupil).
Ipsilateral loss of sweating (face).

It is caused by interruption of sympathetic supply to levator palpebrae superioris and dilator pupillae. This can be caused by lesions in the brain stem, stellate ganglion or root of neck.

Causes
    carcinoma of bronchus (Pancoast tumour)
    syringomyelia (UMN signs in legs, LMN signs in arms)
    syringobulbia (bulbar palsy)
    sympathectomy
    tumour at root of neck, cervical cord.

(4) Large pupil

Causes
    mydriatic drops★
    Holmes–Adie pupil★ (dilated pupil, which responds very slowly to light plus absent ankle jerks in young females)
    third nerve palsy
    surgical (irregular pupil) iridectomy, cataract removal.

(5) Small pupil:

Causes
    old age★
    Horner's syndrome
    pilocarpine† (treatment for glaucoma)
    Argyll Robertson pupil (irregular pupil) with absent light reflex found in syphilis.

(6) Nystagmus

Describe it in terms of the fast phase of movement.

Horizontal nystagmus:

Vestibular causes (associated with deafness and vertigo)
    Meniere's disease
    middle ear surgery
    multiple sclerosis
    syringobulbia
    viral labyrinthitis.

Cerebellar causes (look for other cerebellar signs)
    tumour — primary or secondary
    degenerative disease
    multiple sclerosis
    cerebrovascular disease.

(b) THE CRANIAL NERVES

The examiners may ask you to examine the whole lot, but more often they will select a single cranial nerve for you to examine. This is most often the VIIth cranial nerve (see Table 10.2).

Scheme for examining the cranial nerves

II

Acuity.
Visual fields.   }   See earlier
Fundoscopy.
Pupils: say the afferent arc of the pupillary reflex is lost. This causes an 'afferent pupillary defect'. This is picked up by the 'swinging torch technique'. Swing the torch from pupil to pupil at 1-second intervals: in an afferent pupillary defect the ipsilateral eye will dilate rather than contract when the swinging torch technique is employed.

III, IV, VI (see earlier)

*VII**

Test the facial muscles:

Orbicularis oculi ('screw your eyes up tight and don't let me open them').
Orbicularis ori ('smile, keep your lips together and don't let me open them').
Frontalis muscle ('raise your eyebrows').

This last test distinguishes an upper motor neurone VIIth from a lower motor neurone VIIth lesion. In the latter there is total 'face drop', including frontalis (forehead). In an UMN VIIth nerve lesion the forehead is spared, because of bilateral cortical representation of the frontalis muscle. This is a very commonly asked question.

Summary: UMN VII forehead spared, LMN VII total face drop.

Table 10.2   Cranial nerve palsies

Cranial nerve	Sign	Causes
I‡	Smell (bottles)	Frontal lobe tumour Fractured skull

II	Visual fields
	  scotomata
	  field loss (Fig. 10.2)
	Fundoscopy
	  papillitis
	  optic atrophy
	Pupillary reflexes
	  loss of sensory arc
		MS
		Retro-orbital tumour
		Alcohol
		Tobacco
		Macular degeneration

III†
 	
IV‡
VI†
	Ptosis, large pupil, eye
	  deviation (down and out)
	Diplopia on downward gaze
	Failure of lateral gaze
	  (Fig. 10.1)
		Cavernous sinus thrombosis
		
		Raised intracranial pressure (VI)

V‡ motor sensory	Jaw deviates to side of lesion Anaesthetic area (depends on branch affected) reduced corneal reflex (V^1)	Cerebello-pontine angle tumour

VII*	Ipsilateral face drop
	Bell's sign (LMN only)
		Idiopathic (Bell's palsy)
		Middle ear
		  tumour
		  infection
		Post-surgical
		Sarcoid (sometimes bilateral)

VIII‡	Weber and Rinne tests (see notes)	Wax Otitis media } Otosclerosis } Conductive deafness Trauma Infection VIII nerve } Perceptive deafness tumour } (sensorineural) Streptomycin
IX‡ X XI XII	Uvula deviates away from affected side Reduced bulk of trapezius Reduced power on shrugging shoulders and sternocleidomastoid Ipsilateral wasting of tongue Deviation of tongue to affected side Tongue fasciculation	*Unilateral lesion* Tumour or deposits around jugular foramen *Bilateral lesions* Syringobulbia Motor neurone disease (MND)

Notes about Table 10.3

(1) When examining the VII nerve: if you think it is a LMN lesion, always look behind the ipsilateral ear and over the ipsilateral parotid for scars (mastoid and parotid surgery respectively). These are common causes of this problem, and will make your examination look classy.

(2) Look for Bell's sign (LMN VIIth). On attempted eye closure the ipsilateral eye deviates upwards.

(3) The following can cause any cranial nerve lesion
diabetes
multiple sclerosis (MS)
sarcoid
nerve tumour
post-meningitis.

(4) *Rinne's test.* Hold a tuning fork on the mastoid process until it is no longer audible. Now hold it by the external auditory canal: in the normal ear it should now be audible (air conduction [AC] > bone conduction [BC]). In perceptive deafness (VIIIth nerve problem) this situation persists. In conductive deafness BC > AC because air-conducted sound depends on intact auditory ossicles for its transmission.

(5) *Weber's test.* Place a tuning fork on the vertex of the skull. In normal people it is heard equally well in both ears. In sensory deafness the tuning fork will not be heard in the affected ear. In conductive deafness, the noise will be heard better in the deaf ear. This is because the auditory ossicles are bypassed by direct bone conduction.

(c) SPEECH

(1) Dysarthria

This is a difficulty in the physical articulation of the spoken word caused by a failure of the elements of the 'speech end organ' (i.e. a local cause). There are degrees of dysarthria, and mild dysarthria can be made more pronounced by one of the standard tongue-twisters:

'West Register Street'
'Baby hippopotamus'

Causes
ill-fitting dentures*
cranial nerve palsy VII, IX, X, XII
bulbar palsy
pseudobulbar palsy ('hot potato' speech)
cerebellar disease[†] ('staccato' speech).

Bulbar palsy is caused by bilateral LMN lesions of cranial nerves
IX, X, XII. Patients often complain of nasal regurgitation. Signs
include fasciculating tongue and loss of gag reflex. It is rare and
usually caused by motor neurone disease.

Pseudobulbar palsy is caused by bilateral UMN lesions (e.g. bilateral CVAs). It is more common than a true bulbar palsy. Patients
complain of nasal regurgitation and relatives may say that the patient cries inappropriately (labile emotions). They have a characteristic speech which is high-pitched but rather nasal ('hot potato' or
'Donald Duck' speech). In addition they have a positive jaw jerk
and may have bilateral UMN signs in the limbs.

(2) Dysphasia

There are two types of dysphasia, expressive (or nominal) and
receptive.

In *expressive dysphasia*, which is due to a lesion in Broca's motor
speech area (fronto-parietal), there is a failure of speech content or
expression. This results in the patient being unable to name familiar
objects such as a pen, jacket, etc., whilst knowing what they are.
Its usual cause is a CVA in the dominant hemisphere.

Receptive dysphasia is due to failure of integration of hearing and
speech. This results in the patient being unable to understand the
spoken word. It is usually caused by a CVA or other lesion in
Wernicke's area of the dominant hemisphere (temporo/parietal).

Aphasia is the inability to speak at all.

Patients with both expressive and receptive dysphasia will be unable to name familiar objects. The way to quickly distinguish the
two types of dysphasia is as follows:

Q. 'Can you tell me what this is?' (show the patient a pen)
   Neither will give a meaningful reply.

Q. 'Is it a watch?'
   receptive dysphasic: no meaningful reply.
   expressive dysphasic: 'No!'.

Q. 'Is it a key?'
Receptive dysphasic: no meaningful reply.
Expressive dysphasic: 'No!'.

Q. 'Is it a pen?'
Receptive dysphasic: no meaningful reply.
Expressive dysphasic: 'Yes!'.

(d) HIGHER FUNCTIONS

(1) General cerebral function

Patients with a generalised systemic disease or generalised disease of cerebral substance often have intellectual impairment. You ought to have a list of questions at your fingertips to demonstrate such problems:

Name?
Age?
Address?
Date of birth?
Name of monarch?
Name of prime minister?
Dates of Second World War?
Time?
Recent newsworthy events?
Day of week?
Date?
Place of interview?

Additional tests such as ability to remember three objects, ability to serially subtract 7 from 100 and ability to remember a six figure number can also be valuable. Personally, I have found the name of the current prime minister to be a most valuable question: patients who get this wrong tend to have a very severe cerebral dysfunction.

(2) Frontal lobe function[‡]

Patients with frontal lobe problems tend to be disinhibited. They may wander. They are frequently incontinent. Valuable information is gained from relatives/neighbours.

(3) Parietal lobe function[‡]

On a superficial examination there may be no abnormalities, unless specifically looked for:

Sensory inattention (non-dominant hemisphere).
Apraxia (loss of fine movements associated with a complicated task, e.g. dressing, retrieving a match from a closed matchbox).
Astereognosis (inability to recognise object placed in hand with eyes closed).
Dyslexia (reading difficulties).
Dysgraphia (writing difficulties).
Dyscalculia (mathematical difficulties).
Left/right disorientation.
Finger agnosia.

(2) THE UPPER LIMB

Scheme for the examination of the upper limb

Observation
Wasting.
Fasciculation. } LMN lesions
Posture, e.g. 'waiter's tip', 'claw hand'
Scars, e.g. ulnar nerve transposition.

Tone
Increased (UMN).
Decreased (LMN).
Cogwheel (extrapyramidal).

Power

Root values	Movement
C3, 4	Shoulder abduction
C5, 6	Shoulder adduction
	Elbow flexion
C7	Elbow }
	Wrist } Extension
	Finger }
C8, T1	Small muscles of hand

Peripheral nerve motor supply:

Ulnar: all small muscles of hand with the exception of **LOAF** (median nerve) muscles.
Median:
Lateral two lumbricals (flexion of M/P joints)
Opponens pollicis
Abductor pollicis
Flexor pollicis brevis.
Radial: wrist and finger extensors.

Sensation
Test
  pain (pinprick)
  light touch (cotton wool)
  joint position sense
  vibration (tuning fork).
Temperature sensation is usually irrelevant in the exam.

  You must map out the area of sensory loss and try to deduce whether it is a root or peripheral nerve problem. Remember to compare the sides (see Fig. 10.3 and 10.4 for sensory supply of upper limb).

Reflexes

Reflex	Root
Biceps	C5, 6
Supinator	C6
Triceps	C7, 8

Cerebellar signs
Past pointing.
Intention tremor.
Dysdiadochokinesis.

Involuntary movements
Tremor.
Athetosis.
Chorea.
Ballismus.‡

102 FINAL MB

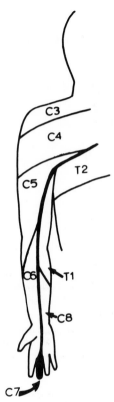

Fig. 10.3 Sensory dermatomes: Upper limbs
C7 is the key to working it out; this supplies middle finger of hand. Note the
C4/T2 interface on the upper chest wall.

TYPICAL CASES

(1) The wasted hand⋆

Very common case.

There are many causes of wasting of the small muscles of the
hand:

Non-neurological
  old age⋆
  rheumatoid arthritis⋆.
Neurological
  cervical rib
  T1 root lesion
  ulnar nerve palsy

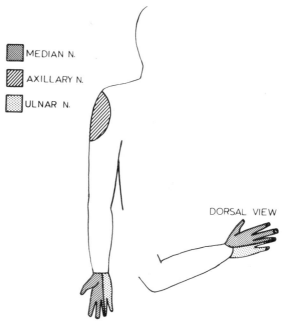

Fig. 10.4 Distribution of sensory loss in peripheral nerve lesions: Upper limbs.
NB: Radial nerve palsies often result in no demonstrable sensory loss
(overlapping nerve supply). Patients sometimes complain of paraesthesiae over
dorsum of thumb.

syringomyelia   ⎫ Often
motor neurone disease. ⎭ bilateral signs

Try to ascertain the cause. Remember that MND and syringomyelia may have UMN signs in the legs. Look for scars around the
elbow (ulnar nerve palsy). It can be difficult to sort out whether it
is a T1 root lesion or an ulnar palsy. Table 10.3 will help.

(2) Ulnar nerve palsy[†]

Usually at the elbow (often traumatic) (see Table 10.3).

Table 10.3   Ulnar nerve and T1 root palsies

	Power	Sensory loss
T1 root	Reduced in all small muscles of hand	Often little
Ulnar nerve	LOAF not affected (median nerve supply)	Inner aspect of medial $1\frac{1}{2}$ fingers and inner aspect of forearm

(3) Median nerve palsy★

Very common.
It will usually be due to carpal tunnel syndrome.

Signs
    reduced power in *LOAF*
    sensory loss lateral $3\frac{1}{2}$ fingers
    Tinel's sign (tapping over median nerve at the wrist causes paraesthesiae).
Causes of carpal tunnel syndrome
    myxoedema
    acromegaly
    rheumatoid arthritis
    pregnancy
    trauma.

It is most common in middle-aged women with none of the above.

(4) Radial nerve palsy[‡]

Rare.
    Wrist drop due to radial nerve palsy (usually) as it passes through the spiral groove. Finger extension and elbow extension are also reduced. It is common in alcoholics and this is the reason for it also being known as 'Saturday night palsy'. After a Saturday night binge, the patient falls sound asleep in the armchair whilst watching TV, his arms having flopped over the edge of the chair. In this position the radial nerve (in the spiral groove) is exposed to trauma from the arm of the chair. Next morning, on awakening, the arm is fairly useless (try to use your own fingers with your wrist fully flexed!), but usually recovers spontaneously.

(5) Nerve to serratus anterior (C5, 6, 7)[‡]

Causes 'winging of the scapula'.

(6) C5, C6 root (Erb-Duchenne palsy)

Causes
    birth trauma
    falling from a motorbike onto the tip of the shoulder.
Signs
    posture—'waiter tip sign' (the arm is held internally rotated with

flexion of the metacarpophalangeal joints)
reduced sensation on outer aspect of the arm
absent biceps and supinator jerks
C5, 6 motor loss (see earlier).

(7) T1 root (Klumpke's palsy)

Causes
  birth trauma
  trauma
  cervical rib
  Pancoast tumour.
Signs
  wasted hand (clawed)
  sensory loss on inner aspect of upper arm.

(8) UMN signs

Unilateral
  e.g. CVA
  cerebral tumour.
Bilateral
  e.g. bilateral CVAs
  MS
  high cord lesion
  syringobulbia
  motor neurone disease (often LMN signs predominate in upper
  limbs).

(9) LMN signs

Unilateral* (see 1-7)
Bilateral[‡]
  syringomyelia
  MND
  bilateral cervical ribs.

(10) Sensory problems[‡]

Sensory signs are usually found in conjunction with motor signs, as
already outlined. It is extremely rare to get a peripheral sensory
neuropathy which solely affects the hands: symptoms in the lower
limbs usually predominate.

(11) Proximal myopathy[‡]

Weakness of proximal muscles. Patients find difficulty in raising their arms (e.g. combing the hair).

Causes
    polymyositis
    dermatomyositis — heliotrope rash under eyes/erythematous rash over hands (50% have an underlying carcinoma)
    Cushing's syndrome
    thyrotoxicosis
    carcinoma
    diabetes
    hereditary.

Don't forget to check the power in the proximal muscles of the legs as these are often affected (inability to stand from the sitting position with the arms folded across the chest).

(12) Parkinson's syndrome (see page 111)

(13) Cerebellar signs (see page 112)

(3) THE LOWER LIMB

Scheme for examination of the lower limb

Use the same routine as that for the upper limb:
Inspection
Wasting.
Scars.
Foot drop, etc.

Tone

Power

Root	Muscle group
L1, 2	Hip flexion
L3, 4	Knee extension
L5, S1	Knee flexion
L4, L5	Ankle dorsiflexion
S1	Ankle plantar flexion

Reflexes
Knee — L3, 4.
Ankle — L5, S1.

Knee and ankle clonus are found in upper motor neurone lesions.

Sensory assessment (see Fig. 10.5)
Remember that sensory dermatomes in the lower limb are rather less clearcut than in the upper limbs.

Coordination
Heel/shin test.

Romberg's test

Gait (see page 110)

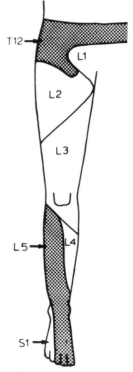

Fig. 10.5   Sensory dermatomes: lower limbs.

TYPICAL CASES

(1) Sensory neuropathy*

Common case.

Symmetrical sensation loss.
All modalities affected.
'Glove and stocking' distribution, but lower limbs affected first and more severely.
Causes
   alcohol*
   diabetes*
   carcinomatosis*
   drugs[†] (e.g. nitrofurantoin)
   vitamin deficiency[†] (especially the B group).

Rare causes: Guillan–Barre syndrome, amyloid, sarcoid, uraemia, myeloma, porphyria, leprosy.

Remember to look for the consequences of neuropathy, e.g.

   Painless ulcers.
   Charcot's joints (ankle, knee).

(2) Foot drop[†]

Lateral peroneal nerve palsy. It is often caused by trauma to the head of the fibula (bumper-bar injury) but can be found spontaneously in diabetics.

Signs
   foot drop
   high stepping gait on affected side
   sensory examination ⎫
   reflexes. ⎬ Normal
Other causes of foot drop
   mononeuritis multiplex
   peripheral neuropathy
   motor neurone disease
   peroneal muscular atrophy (Charcot–Marie–Tooth syndrome).

(3) Root lesion[‡]

L5

Weakness of extensors of the great toe.

Reduced/absent ankle jerk.
Reduced sensation over L5 dermatome.

S1

Reduced power
  plantar flexion
  foot eversion.
Absent ankle jerk.
Reduced sensation over outer aspect of foot.

L2–4

These root lesions are very rare.

Causes
  prolapsed intervertebral disc*
  metastases‡
  meningioma.

(4) Unilateral UMN signs*

Found in common-or-garden cerebrovascular accidents.

(5) Bilateral UMN signs (spastic paraparesis)

Rare in practice, common in examinations.

Signs
  bilateral
    hypertonia
    hyper-reflexia
    plantar extensors
    ankle/knee clonus
    weakness
    sensory loss.

You *must* look for a 'sensory level' (use a pin on abdominal and thoracic walls). This will tell you the level of the lesion in the spinal cord.

Causes
  trauma (usually RTA)
  vertebral collapse
    metastatic cancer
    osteoporosis

tumours
  extradural
    meningioma
    angioma
    neurofibroma
    metastases
  intrinsic
    e.g. glioma
spinal artery embolism
multiple sclerosis
motor neurone disease
syringomyelia/bulbia.

(6) Charcot–Marie–Tooth Disease[‡]

Peroneal muscular atrophy.
  Rare case.
  Autosomal dominant condition causing wasting of peroneal muscles in early adult life. Eventually all the lower leg muscles waste causing the 'inverted champagne bottle' appearance.

Signs
  wasting
  foot drop
  impaired vibration sense and general sensory loss
  signs in the upper limbs (very rare).

(4) ABNORMAL GAITS AND MOVEMENTS

(a) ABNORMAL GAITS

(1) Cerebrovascular accident (CVA)[†]

There is a rigid leg and partially plantar flexed foot. The patient drags his leg through a semicircle.

(2) Spastic paraplegia

The patient drags both spastic legs. He usually swings the upper torso to help him move. This has been described as a 'wading through mud gait'.

(3) Dorsal column loss

The patient looks at the ground. He has a wide-based gait with high foot lift. The patient will fall if the eyes are closed (Romberg's sign).

Other signs
   loss of joint position and vibration sense
Causes
   diabetes
   Friedreich's ataxia
   subacute combined degeneration of the cord
   tabes dorsalis.

(4) Foot drop gait

High stepping gait.
Feet slap the ground.
Causes
   lateral peroneal nerve palsy
   poliomyelitis
   Charcot–Marie–Tooth disease
   motor neurone disease.

(5) Proximal myopathy

Waddling gait (looks like a duck). The upper torso swings to aid forward propulsion of the limbs. The patient will have difficulty getting out of a chair (see earlier).

(6) Parkinson's disease[†]

Shuffling gait. Small steps. The patient is stooped and rigid, and finds turning difficult. The arms do not swing. Festination (sudden increase in speed of walking). On/off phenomenon — (patient suddenly 'freezes' during a movement — a most distressing symptom). Patients with Parkinson's disease find initiating movements difficult.

   Remember to assess how the patient's illness affects his daily life, e.g. dressing (buttons may be impossible), eating, etc.
Other signs
   (a) tremor
       6 Hz

    pill rolling
    better during voluntary action
  (b) bradykinesia
      facial immobility
  (c) rigidity.
Causes
  idiopathic
  drugs, e.g. major tranquillisers
  vascular (multiple CVAs to the basal ganglia). This variety is usually unresponsive to therapy
  post-viral (encephalitis lethargia occurred in the early 1920s— most of these patients are now dead).

(7) Cerebellar disease

Gait: veering
  Patients fall to side of the lesion (this is accentuated by asking the patient to walk along an imaginary white line on the floor).
Other signs (all ipsilateral)
  dysarthria
  nystagmus (fast phase to side of lesion)
  intention tremor (this is an oscillating tremor worse on movement)
  past pointing (finger nose test)
  dysdiadochokinesis
  poor heel/shin test
  cerebellar drift (when the patient holds his hands outstretched there is ipsilateral upward drift or oscillation)
  hypotonia
  hyporeflexia.
Causes
  CVA★
    haemorrhage
    infarction
  tumour
    secondary★
    primary‡
    non-metastatic degeneration (with carcinoma of the bronchus)
  degenerative
    multiple sclerosis†
    alcoholism†

familial, e.g. Friedreich's ataxia
hypothyroidism‡

Note. Lesions of the cerebellar vermis (central part of the cerebellum) cause a peculiar sign called truncal ataxia. This results in instability and writhing movements of the upper torso, accentuated by asking the patient to sit forwards with his arms folded.

(b) ABNORMAL MOVEMENTS

(1) Tremor

Resting
   physiological★ (worse with alcohol)
   Parkinson's disease★
   benign essential tremor (better with alcohol, often familial)
   Wilson's disease

Note. Treatment with β_2 agonists and thyrotoxicosis cause an exaggerated physiological tremor.

Worse on movement
   cerebellar tremor† (intention tremor)

Note: Severe parkinsonian and benign essential tremors are sometimes worse on movement.

(2) Chorea

Causes
   drugs, e.g. L-dopa
   CVA (basal ganglia)‡
   tumour (basal ganglia)‡
   Sydenham's chorea
   thyrotoxicosis
   SLE.

(3) Athetosis

Causes
   cerebral palsy★
   post-cerebral anoxia† (e.g. cardiac arrest, drowning, etc)
   Wilson's disease
   hereditary.

(4) Hemiballismus[‡]

Ipsilateral lesion to subthalamic nucleus.
Responds to chlorpromazine.

(5) DIFFUSE NEUROLOGICAL DISEASE

Many neurological diseases cut across artificial anatomical boundaries. Be prepared to ask to examine other aspects of the nervous system, if you think this is relevant.

(1) CVA★

This causes a pyramidal weakness in both the upper and lower limb, if the lesion involves the cerebral cortex, internal capsule, or pyramidal tracts as they run through the brain stem.

It is important to know the classical distribution of a pyramidal motor weakness.

The weak muscle groups are:

Shoulder abduction.
Elbow and wrist extension.
Finger abduction.
Hip flexors.
Hamstrings.
Dorsiflexion of foot.

The easy way to remember this is to recall the typical posture of a stroke victim, due to the stronger, intact (spastic) muscle groups.

The arm is adducted at the shoulder and flexed at the elbow and wrist. The leg is held straight and the foot drags on walking, due to intact glutei, quadriceps and plantar flexors.

If you find a pyramidal weakness in one leg it is important to examine the ipsilateral arm and controlateral leg for signs of pyramidal weakness. This is because the causes of a spastic hemiparesis and a spastic paraparesis are quite different (see earlier).

(2) Multiple sclerosis★

This is a diffuse demyelinating process of unknown aetiology. It commonly starts in early adult life and affects women more frequently than men. It seems to be more common in temperate zones. Spontaneous relapses and remissions occur, but there is usually a gradual overall deterioration through the years. Patients commonly end up wheelchair-bound in the later stages of the disease.

The signs will depend on the sites involved and the stage of the disease:

UMN deficit
  hemiparesis
  paraparesis
  monoparesis.
Cerebellar signs
  often bilateral
  ataxic nystagmus (pathognomonic). = INTERNULLEAR OPHTHALMOPLEGIA
Optic atrophy.
Sensory disturbances.
III, IV or VI nerve palsies.
Painless retention of urine.
Cerebral cortex involvement — inappropriate euphoria is frequently seen in the later stages of the disease.

(3) Motor neurone disease

Exceptionally rare in clinical practice. Not quite so rare in exams. There is a progressive, idiopathic degeneration of the anterior horn cells (spinal cord), cranial nerve nuclei and pyramidal tracts. There are *no* sensory signs.

There are three patterns of neurological signs, but there is often overlap between these groups.

(i) True bulbar palsy (see earlier)

Bilateral cranial nerve palsies of IX–XII.

(ii) Progressive muscular atrophy

Bilateral degeneration of the anterior horn cells. This causes bilateral lower motor neurone signs in the hands, followed by the feet. There is prominent muscle fasciculation. Loss of deep tendon reflexes.

(iii) Amyotrophic lateral sclerosis

Pyramidal tract degeneration.
Spastic paraparesis. Arms usually affected later (and less extensively).

(4) Syringomyelia[‡]

Cyst in cervical spinal cord (anterior position). It presents in early adult life and slowly progresses over 20 years.
The cyst encroaches on tracts which lie anteriorly:

Lateral spinothalamic (pain and temperature).
Anterior horn cells (LMN).
Pyramidal (UMN).

Signs
dissociated sensory loss (arms)
painless lesions in the upper limbs
Charcot's joints (wrist, elbow)
wasting of the small muscles of the hand
UMN signs in the legs.

(5) Syringobulbia[‡]

Same as syringomyelia, but the lesion is in the lower brain stem/upper cervical cord.
Signs are very similar, but in addition there may be

Ipsilateral V nerve palsy.   ⎫ Involvement of cranial
Bulbar palsy.   ⎭ nerve nuclei
Ipsilateral Horner's syndrome (cervical sympathetic nerves).
Nystagmus (brain stem cerebellar connections).

KEY QUESTIONS

(1) What are the causes of
     (i) ptosis?
    (ii) VI nerve palsy?
   (iii) XII nerve palsy?
   (iv) pseudobulbar palsy?
    (v) anosmia?
   (vi) wasting of the hand?
  (vii) carpal tunnel syndrome?
 (viii) proximal myopathy?
   (ix) parkinsonism?
    (x) sensory neuropathy?
   (xi) spastic paraparesis?
  (xii) dorsal column loss?
 (xiii) cerebellar disease?
 (xiv) resting tremor?

(2) Which muscles of the hand are served by the median nerve?

(3) What are the causes of an absent red reflex?

(4) What is Romberg's sign?
What is its significance?

(5) What are the neurological manifestations of the acquired immune-deficiency syndrome?

(6) What is the difference, on clinical examination, between an ulnar nerve palsy and a T1 root lesion?

11 Rheumatology

Rheumatological cases are common in MB because rheumatological disease is common, often resulting in chronic physical signs.

Scheme for examination of the joints

Look — Feel — Move

(1) Inspection

General. Start by observing the patient generally. Active attention to this point may give you the diagnosis immediately, e.g.

Butterfly rash on face (SLE).
Small mouth, beaked nosed (scleroderma).
Stooped posture (ankylosing spondylitis).
Scaly rash (psoriatic arthropathy).

Joints. Now concentrate on the joint(s) in question. The examiner will tell you which joint(s) he wishes you to examine. Look at the joints from the front, back and sides. In particular you are looking for:

Swelling.
Erythema.
Joint deformity.
Scars (previous surgery).

(2) Palpation

Always ask the patient if the joint(s) are tender — if they are you must palpate carefully. Try not to hurt the patient (keep glancing at his face).

Look for:

Tenderness.
Synovial thickening.
Joint effusion.
Deformity.
Associated muscle wasting.

(3) Movement

Passive. Move the patient's joint (gently) to assess its range in all directions of normal movement. Again, be careful, it is easy to hurt the patient.

Active. Now ask the patient to move the joint himself in the same modalities.

Functional movement. Try to get an idea of how the patient's joint disease has affected that joint's function, e.g.

Hip joint
  ask the patient to walk, stand from the sitting position.
Hand
  grip
  thumb opposition
  writing
  use of knife and fork
  buttoning a shirt, etc.

(4) Further aspects of examination

As directed by your findings.

Always look for rheumatoid nodules on the elbows. Also look for:

Nail changes. } psoriatic
Skin lesions. } arthropathy
Gouty tophi (ear, periarticular).
Scleroderma facies/skin.
Nailfold telangiectasia (SLE, RA).
Butterfly rash (SLE).

TYPICAL CASES

(1) Rheumatoid arthritis (RA)*

Most commonly you are presented with a pair of arthritic hands. Often, with end-stage disease, the diagnosis is obvious. Occasionally you are presented with more acute joints. This is more difficult. The diagnosis may not be immediately obvious, and there is a risk of hurting the patient. If the skin overlying a joint is erythematous proceed with caution.

Signs

Hands (see Plates 6a and b)
    swelling
    erythema
    synovial thickening/tenderness
    wasting of the small muscles of the hand
    deformity, e.g. metacarpophalangeal subluxation
    ulnar deviation
    swan neck deformity ⎫
    Boutonniere deformity ⎬ See Fig.11.1
    'Z' deformity of the thumb ⎭
    Reduced function.

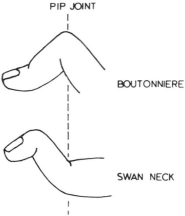

Fig. 11.1 Finger deformities: rheumatoid arthritis.

---

* Very common.
† Common.
‡ Rare and/or difficult.

Always look for rheumatoid nodules (Plate 6b).

Ask about other affected joints.

Rheumatoid arthritis usually, but not always, affects joints symmetrically. In the hand the proximal joints, e.g. the metacarpophalangeal joints (MCP) and the proximal interphalangeal (PIP) joint are predominantly affected. RA is much more common in females.

Complications of RA

RA is a systemic disease and the complications include:

Sjogren's syndrome
  dry eyes
  dry mouth
  arthritis.
Episcleritis.
Fibrosing alveolitis.
Caplan's syndrome (rheumatoid lung nodules with associated pneumoconiosis).
Pericarditis.
Vasculitis (vasculitic leg ulcers and mononeuritis multiplex).
Sensory neuropathy
Felty's syndrome
  RA
  splenomegaly
  pancytopenia.
Amyloidosis (causes renal failure).
Anaemia (of chronic disorders).

(2) **Systemic Lupus Erythematosus**[†]

Much more common in women.
Onset early 20s.

Signs

Arthritis
  usually symmetrical, often migratory
  affects the hands, wrists, elbows, knees and ankles.
Skin
  photosensitivity

    butterfly rash
    Raynaud's phenomenon
    arteritic lesions
    alopecia.
Sjogren's syndrome.
Lung
    alveolitis (crackles both sides)
    pleural effusion.
Heart
    pericarditis (rub)
    myocarditis
    Libman–Sachs endocarditis.
Kidneys
    proteinuria
    nephrotic syndrome
    chronic renal failure.
Nervous system
    cerebral lupus
      confusion
      intellectual impairment
      pyschiatric symptoms
    mononeuritis multiplex
    peripheral neuropathy.

(3) Scleroderma[†]

More common in females.

Signs

Skin
    tightened skin which is shiny, with loss of hair and pigmentation.
    (Try to pick up the skin on the back of the patient's hand between
    your thumb and index finger. This will be impossible.)
    telangiectasia
    facial appearance
      tight skin
      beaked nose
      microstomia
    Raynaud's phenomenon.
Chest
    alveolitis (basal crackles).

Heart
   pericarditis (rub)
   congestive cardiac failure.
Gut
   oesophageal involvement (dysphagia)
   small bowel involvement (malabsorption).
Arthritis
   small joints of the hand (usually).
Renal
   chronic renal failure $\pm$ hypertension.

(4) Ankylosing Spondylitis[†]

Much more common in men.
   It usually presents in the 20s or 30s.
   Over 95% are HLA B27+ve.

Signs

Fixed spine
   thoracic kyphosis
   loss of lumbar lordosis
   hyperextension of neck (this results in the typical 'question mark'
   posture — see Plate 7).
Arthritis
   large joint monoarthritis of the lower limb
   sacroileitis (pelvis 'spring').

X-ray

Poor chest expansion.
Bamboo spine.
Sacroileitis.

Associations

Aortic regurgitation.
Iritis, conjunctivitis.
Pulmonary fibrosis (apical).
Mycetoma[‡] (fungus ball in under-aerated upper lobe).

Sacroileitis may also be found in inflammatory bowel disease.

(5) Psoriatic arthropathy

M = F.

Signs

Arthritis (there are three main patterns of joint involvement)
  terminal interphalangeal joints (distinguishes it from RA), usually asymmetrical
  polyarthropathy indistinguishable from RA, but seronegative
  arthritis mutilans — resorption of phalangeal heads resulting in a destructive arthropathy of the hands.
Skin
  psoriatic plaques
  pitting of fingernails
  onycholysis
  scaling of scalp.

There are no rheumatoid nodules as this is a seronegative arthritis. The skin changes may be minimal.

Remember that RA and psoriasis are common; not every patient with arthritis and psoriasis will have psoriatic arthropathy. These two conditions can coexist (see Plates 8a and b).

(6) Gout

(a) Chronic gout[†]

Chronic elevation of serum urate.

Signs

Gouty tophi
  periarticular
  pinna of ear.
Arthritis
  osteoarthrosis (OA) of the affected joints.

(b) Acute gout[‡]

Signs

Arthritis (asymmetrical).
Great toe.

Wrist/elbow.
Any other joint may be affected.

Causes

Idiopathic.
Thiazide diuretics.
Renal failure.
Psoriasis.
Myeloproliferative disorders.

(7) Monoarthritis

Causes

Trauma.
Sepsis
   bacterial (including tuberculosis and gonorrhoea)
   viral, e.g. rubella.
Seronegative arthritides
   osteoarthrosis (OA)
   psoriasis
   ankylosing spondylitis (hip, knee)
   Reiter's disease (ankle, knee)
   gout
   pseudogout (knee).

RA (monoarthritis is an unusual but recognised mode of presentation).
SLE, scleroderma.
Crohn's disease, ulcerative colitis (hip, knee, ankle).

(8) Raynaud's phenomenon

Signs

May be none (history important).
Dystrophic changes.
Loss of the fingertips.   Severe
Nail changes.   cases
Frank digital gangrene.   only

Causes

Raynaud's disease (idiopathic).
Scleroderma.
RA, SLE.
Cervical rib.
Atherosclerotic.
Polycythaemia.

It is more common in people who use vibrating tools.
Remember to look for scars in the root of the neck indicating that the patient has had a sympathectomy to alleviate the symptoms.

KEY QUESTIONS

(1) What are the causes of
    (i) Raynaud's phenomenon?
    (ii) sacroileitis?
    (iii) gout?
    (iv) monoarthritis of the ankle?
(2) What are the differences radiologically between rheumatoid arthritis and osteoarthritis?
(3) What are the systemic complications of rheumatoid arthritis?
(4) What is Reiter's syndrome?

12 Anatomical considerations: the upper limb, the lower limb, the face

You may be asked to examine part of the patient's anatomy, with no specific clues from the examiner as to which system contains the abnormal physical sign. This can wrong-foot the unwary candidate unless you specifically prepare yourself in advance.

The three commonest areas asked about are:

(1) The upper limb.
(2) The lower limb.
(3) The face.

The question may be:
'Examine this patient's hands.' or
'Look at this patient's face.'
You will realise that, because of basic anatomical considerations, you will more than likely find the abnormality in the skin, nervous system or joints. Your examination should be tailored accordingly. Remember to inspect carefully. This may tell you where to concentrate your examination, or give you the diagnosis immediately. Don't forget to examine the peripheral pulses when examining the limbs.

(1) The upper limb

If you are presented with an upper limb think of

Skin.
Joints.
Nervous system.

Skin

Psoriasis.

Eczema.
Lichen planus.
Scleroderma, etc. (see Chapter 9).

Joints

RA (rheumatoid nodules).
OA (Heberden's nodes).
Gout.
SLE.
Psoriatic arthropathy (see Chapter 11).

Nervous system.

For example:
Wasted hand.
Ulnar nerve lesion.
Median nerve lesion.
Tremor (see Chapter 10).

Miscellaneous

Look particularly carefully at the hand for signs of:

Clubbing (Chapter 5).
Palmar erythema (Chapter 6)
Nail changes
   pits
   onycholysis   } (Chapter 9)
   nailfold infarction.
Dupuytren's contracture.
Raynaud's phenomenon (Chapter 11).

(2) The lower limb

Skin

Leg ulcers★.
Psoriasis, dermatitis, etc (Chapter 9).
Pyoderma gangrenosum‡
Ulcer on lower limb with raised purple edge (irregular) and necrotic base. It is associated with RA and inflammatory bowel disease.

Pretibial myxoedema[‡]
 pink/skin-coloured induration, areas of which have a *'peau d'orange'* appearance. This is found over the shins in thyrotoxicosis (very rare). There is sometimes an associated hypertrichosis.

Necrobiosis lipoidica[‡]
 Oval indurated plaques found on the shins of diabetics (rare). The plaques have brownish margins and yellow waxy areas of atrophy.

Joints

RA.
OA.
Gout.
SLE (Chapter 11).

Nervous system

For example:

Peripheral neuropathy.
Charcot joint (see Plate 9).
Spastic monoparesis.
Spastic paraparesis, etc. (Chapter 10).

Miscellaneous

Swollen lower legs
 peripheral oedema
  CCF
  hypoproteinaemia.
 deep venous thrombosis ⎫
 ruptured Baker's cyst. ⎬ Unilateral
Absent peripheral pulses
 peripheral arterial disease.

(3) The face

Rheumatological diseases are much less common. Endocrinological disorders are more important.

Skin

Psoriasis, dermatitis, etc.
Acne, rosacea etc.
SLE (butterfly rash).
Scleroderma (beaked nose, microstomia, tight skin).
Malar flush (mitral valve disease).
Flushing (carcinoid syndrome).
Suffusion. ⎫
Oedema.   ⎬ SVC obstruction
Herpes zoster.
Alopecia.
Lupus pernio (sarcoid of nose, which is large and red/purple).
Rhinophyma (rosacea affecting nose, which is large and blue/red).
Xanthelasmata (hyperlipidaemia).
Dermatomyositis (heliotrope colour of eyelids).
Hereditary haemorrhagic telangiectasis; telangiectasiae around mouth, lips and gums; associated with GI bleeding. Autosomal dominant.
Peutz–Jeghers syndrome: perioral lentiginoses (brown spots) associated with benign small bowel tumours. Autosomal dominant.

Nervous system (Chapter 10)

Cranial nerve palsies.
Eye signs.
Parkinsonian facies.
Tardive dyskinesia (phenothiazines).

Endocrine system (Chapter 8)

Hypothyroidism.
Hyperthyroidism.
Acromegaly.
Cushing's syndrome.

Miscellaneous

Paget's disease (frontal bossing).
Saddle nose (syphilis, Wegener's granulomatosis).
Senile arcus.
Anaemia. ⎫
Jaundice. ⎬ Chapter 6

Parotid swelling
  tumour
  cirrhosis
  Sjogren's syndrome
  mumps
  sarcoid
  lymphoma.

13 The electrocardiogram (ECG)

You need to have a basic grasp of the ECG: you ought to be able to recognise simple abnormalities, e.g. myocardial infarction. Some medical schools specifically exclude ECG diagnosis from their clinical paper (I am not sure why). It is worthwhile finding out what emphasis is placed on ECGs in the exam you are sitting and tailoring your revision accordingly.

(1) READING THE ECG

Look at each individual part of the ECG in turn, using the following list:

Rate.
Rhythm.
Axis.
P wave.
PR interval.
QRS complex.
ST segment.
T wave.
U wave.
Pattern recognition.

Like most things in medicine it is best to start off with a routine and adhere rigidly to it, at least in the first instance. Look at as many ECGs as possible and read them using this scheme. You will eventually reach a point (perhaps in years to come) when a glance will be sufficient to tell you the diagnosis (by pattern recognition). Do not do this in the examination.

Note: On most ECGs with standard settings: one small square (1 mm) = 0.04 s; one large square (5 mm) = 0.2 s.

(1) Rate

Simple. Measure the distance (in large squares) between two consecutive R waves and divide into 300, that is:

$$\frac{300}{\text{R–R interval}}$$

For example, if R–R interval is four squares:

$$\text{Rate} = \frac{300}{4} = 75 \text{ beats/min}$$

Bradycardia: rate < 60, tachycardia: rate > 100.

(2) Rhythm

This can be rather more tricky. Having said this I think it would be unfair for you to be shown a complex arrhythmia.

(a) Normal sinus rhythm

There is a P wave before each QRS complex.
    PR interval < 0.2 s (five small squares).
    QRS complex width < 0.12 s (three small squares).

(b) Ectopics (Fig. 13.1)

Ventricular. The QRS complex is wide (< 0.12 s) and bizarre in shape.

Atrial. The P wave is an unusual shape, or may be inverted. It will come slightly earlier or slightly later than expected. The QRS complex is normal width.

(c) Tachyarrhythmias

Supraventricular. The width of the QRS complex is normal (i.e. < 0.12 s) and the rate >100 beats/min.

  (i) Sinus tachycardia
       P wave before each QRS complex R-R interval regular.
  (ii) Supraventricular tachycardia
       aetiology uncertain — regular R–R interval
       P waves may not be evident, e.g. nodal tachycardia, atrial tachycardia.

P WAVE ABNORMALITIES

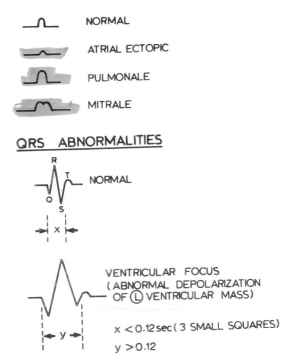

NORMAL

ATRIAL ECTOPIC

PULMONALE

MITRALE

QRS ABNORMALITIES

NORMAL

VENTRICULAR FOCUS
(ABNORMAL DEPOLARIZATION
OF Ⓛ VENTRICULAR MASS)

x < 0.12 sec (3 SMALL SQUARES)
y > 0.12

Fig. 13.1 P wave and QRS abnormalities.

(iii) Atrial fibrillation
no P waves
irregularly irregular R–R interval
irregular fibrillating pattern of baseline. — *Esp* V_1

Ventricular
(i) *Ventricular tachycardia* (VT)
broad complex (QRS > 0.12 s)
tachyarrhythmia (rate > 100 beats/min)
P wave impossible to see (usually).
Occasionally atrial beats can be conducted to the ventricles
through an abnormal pathway at the a-v node. This can
cause an SVT with aberrant conduction, which may be
indistinguishable from VT. (This is postgraduate medicine.)
(ii) *Ventricular fibrillation* (VF). Bizarre waveform with no
discernible baseline or meaningful complexes. The patient

will have no output ('cardiac arrest'). If the patient has a pulse then check the ECG leads, as one has probably fallen off.

(d) Bradyarrhythmias

(i) Sinus bradycardia
P waves are present and regular
rate < 60 beats/min
normal QRS configuration.

(ii) Nodal
— no p waves at all
— rate < 60 beats/min
— normal QRS configuration.

(iii) Heart block (Fig. 13.2).

This is caused by an increased refractory period of the a-v node (of varying degrees of severity). In complete heart block the a-v node will allow no electrical impulse to pass from the atria to the ventricles, which therefore function independently.

First degree (1°)
PR interval > 0.2 s. all P waves followed by normal QRS.

Second degree (2°)
Wenckebach (Mobitz type I). PR interval gradually increases in length until there is a dropped beat (atrial beat not transmitted to ventricles via a-v node).

Mobitz type II. PR interval 0.2 s. Dropped beats (a-v conduction failure) are regular: e.g. two to one block (2 : 1) — alternate beats dropped; three to one block (3 : 1) — every third beat dropped. Mobitz type II has a more serious prognosis, as it often progresses to complete heart block.

Complete heart block (3°)
Complete a-v dissociation.
P waves bear no relationship to QRS.
QRS may be wide and bizarre-shaped. The rate may drop very low (20 beats/min). This causes reduced cardiac output and syncope.

(3) Axis

Easy, if you know how.
Use the diagram of electrical vectors (Fig. 13.3) and the standard leads (I, II, III, AVF, AVL, AVR) of Case 1.

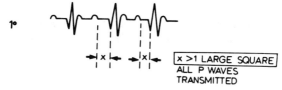

1°

x >1 LARGE SQUARE
ALL P WAVES
TRANSMITTED

2° a) WENCKEBACH (MOBITZ TYPE I)

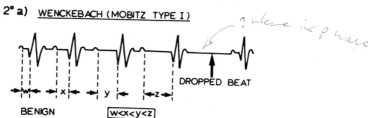

↑ where is P wave

DROPPED BEAT

BENIGN

w<x<y<z

2°b) MOBITZ TYPE II

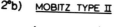

P WAVES

2:1 BLOCK
MAY PROGRESS TO COMPLETE HEART BLOCK

3° COMPLETE HEART BLOCK

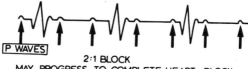

P WAVES

COMPLETE A/V DISSOCIATION
P WAVES BEAR NO RELATIONSHIP
TO QRS COMPLEXES

Fig. 13.2 Heart block.

Find the *isoelectric lead* (i.e. the one in which the size of the R wave is most equivalent to the size of the S wave.) In Case 1 it is lead AVF.

Check this against the diagram of electrical vectors (Fig. 13.3). In this instance the isoelectric vector will be at approximately + 90°. Now look at the ECG again and find the lead(s) with the greatest positive deflection (i.e. the largest R waves). In Case 1, this is I and AVL.

The electrical axis of the heart will be at 90° to the isoelectric lead in the direction of the large R waves

Electrical axis (Case 1) = 0°
Normal axis ranges from + 90° to −30°.

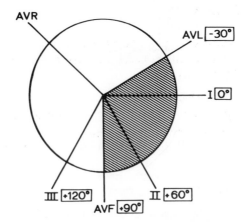

Fig. 13.3 Electrical axis. The shaded area represents the normal range of electrical axis.

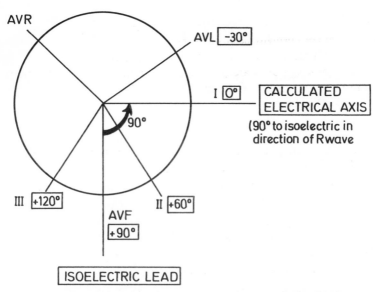

Fig. 13.4 Working out the electrical axis. The calculation of electrical axis in this diagram refers to the ECG of case 1, to be found later in this Chapter.

(4) P wave (Fig. 13.1)

It should be less than 2.5 mm (small squares).
It is tallest in lead II and it is for this reason that lead II is often used as the rhythm strip.

'P' mitrale (mitral valve disease)
    double-topped P wave due to left atrial enlargement.
'P' pulmonale (pulmonary hypertension)
    large single-peaked P wave due to right atrial enlargement.

(5) PR interval

From the start of the P wave to the start of the R wave should be 0.12–0.2 s (3–5 small squares).

PR > 0.2 = first-degree heart block.
PR < 0.12 is seen in the re-entrant tachycardias, e.g. Wolff–Parkinson–White syndrome.

(6) QRS complex

Q waves

Q waves are normally seen in AVR.
They are sometimes seen in III in normal individuals.
Pathological Q waves are greater than 1 mm × 1 mm and denote transmural infarction of the myocardium.

R waves

The R wave should get bigger as you go across the V leads, V1–6.
There is often little or no R wave in V1.
    Causes of large R wave in V1:

Dextrocardia.
Pulmonary embolus.
Right ventricular hypertrophy.
Wolff–Parkinson–White (type A).
True posterior myocardial infarction.

In Wolff–Parkinson–White syndrome (W–P–W) the R wave has a slurred upstroke (delta wave) due to abnormal conduction of im-

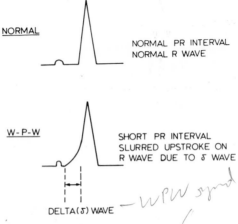

Fig. 13.5 The delta wave.

pulses through the a-v node via an aberrant pathway (see Fig. 13.5). These patients are prone to tachyarrhythmias such as atrial fibrillation.

S wave

The S wave should get smaller as you traverse the V leads (V1–V6).

Bundle branch block (BBB)

Here the QRS complex is wide (> 0.12 s). In right BBB the QRS complex will be mainly upright in V1 and V2.

In left BBB the QRS complex will be mainly upright in leads V5 and 6. LBBB makes the rest of the ECG uninterpretable. (see 'Typical cases').

(7) ST segment

This should be normally at the same level as the baseline.

Raised ST segment

Convex upwards
  acute myocardial infarction
  some normal negroes.

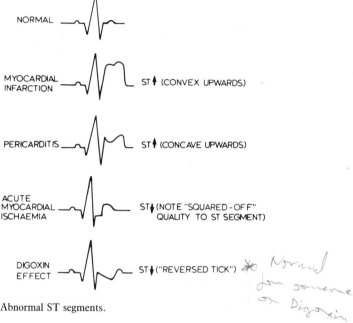

Fig. 13.6   Abnormal ST segments.

Concave upwards
    pericarditis (especially in leads V5, 6, I and AVL).

Depressed ST segment

Acute myocardial ischaemia.
Digoxin effect (see Fig. 13.6).

Note: The 'digoxin effect' does not imply digoxin toxicity, but simply that the patient is currently taking digoxin.

(8) T wave

Peaked T wave

Myocardial ischaemia.
Hyperkalaemia.

Peaked T waves are occasionally seen in the very early stages of acute myocardial infarction.

Inverted T wave

Myocardial ischaemia.
Post-myocardial infarction.
Hypokalaemia.
Left ventricular hypertrophy/strain.
Following bundle branch block pattern.

U waves

Seen after the T wave as a little blip on the baseline.

Causes
    normal fit young adults
    myocardial ischaemia
    hypokalaemia.

(10) Pattern Recognition

Essentially this means synthesising all the information you have
gleaned from going through the above scheme. You should try to
fit all the abnormalities together to make a diagnosis.

Experts can glance at an ECG and make an immediate diagnosis.
This comes from years of practice perfecting their pattern recognition skills. You may find such people rather irritating — don't
worry, you will be able to do it in the end, it's just a matter of
enough practice.

(2) TYPICAL CASES

This section gives you a chance to read specimen ECGS, similar to
the ones you may be presented with during the examination. I suggest that you read them in the way I have demonstrated. The
answers are to be found on the following page.

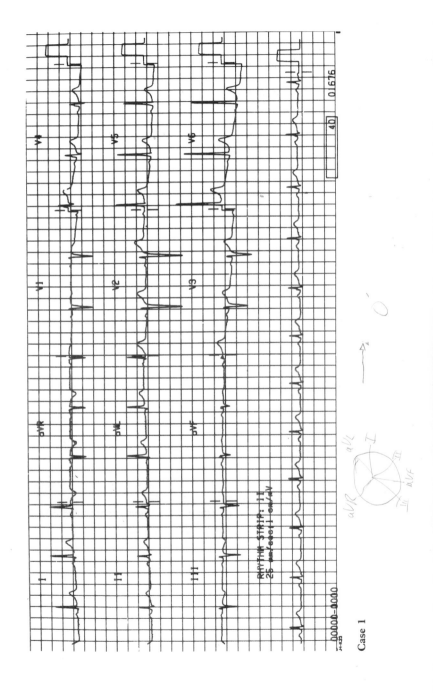

Case 1

Case 1

Rate:	75/min
Rhythm:	Sinus rhythm
Axis:	0°
P wave:	Normal
PR interval:	0.12 s
QRS complex:	Normal
ST segment:	Normal
T waves:	Normal
	Note inverted T waves in V1, AVR and III. This is normal
U waves:	Absent
Pattern recognition:	Normal ECG

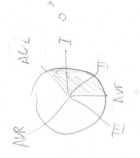

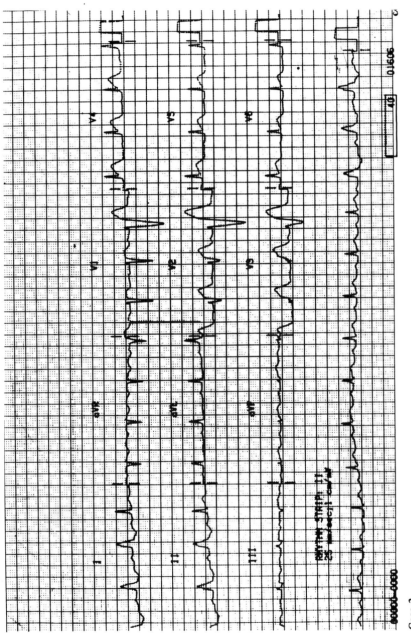

Case 2

Case 2

Rate:	80/min
Rhythm:	Sinus
Axis:	0°
P wave:	Normal
PR interval:	0.2 s (upper limit of normal)
QRS complex:	One ventricular ectopic (V1–3)
	Broad-looking complexes I, II
ST segment:	Raised V2–6
T wave:	Prominent V2–5
U wave:	Absent
Pattern recognition:	Acute anterior myocardial infarction

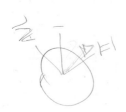

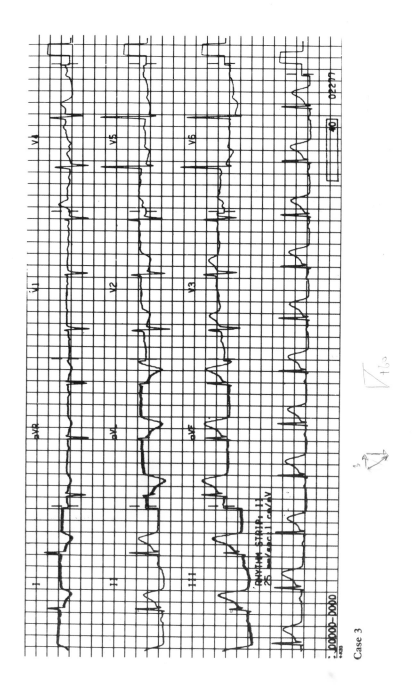

Case 3

Case 3

Rate:	70/min
Rhythm:	Sinus
Axis:	+60°
P wave:	Normal
PR interval:	0.16 s
QRS:	Normal
ST segment:	Raised ST II, III, AVF
	Depressed ST V5, 6, I, AVL
T wave:	Inverted V4–6, I, AVL
U wave:	Present V4–6
Pattern recognition:	Acute inferior myocardial infarction, with associated anterolateral myocardial ischaemia

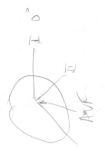

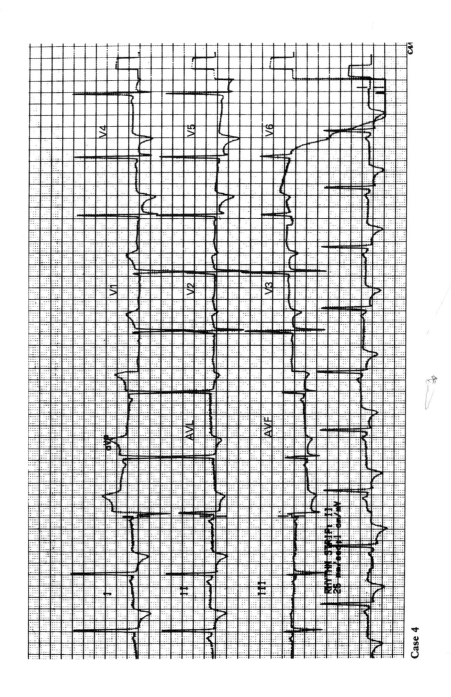

Case 4

Case 4

Rate:	60/min
Rhythm:	Sinus
Axis:	+15°
P wave:	Normal
PR interval:	0.12 s
QRS complex:	Large R waves V2–6, I, II
	Deep S waves V1–3
	R wave V5 + S wave V1 = 49 mm
ST segment:	Widespread depression
T wave:	Inverted V2–6, I, II, AVL, AVF
U wave:	Absent
Pattern recognition:	Left ventricular hypertrophy

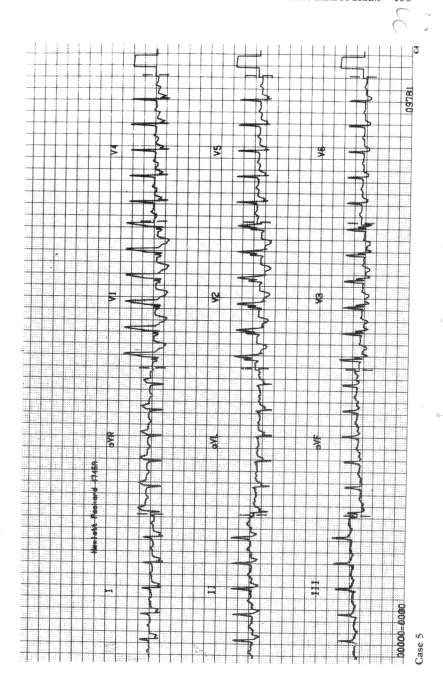

Case 5

Case 5

Rate:	150/min
Rhythm:	Atrial fibrillation
Axis:	+ 90°
P wave:	Absent
QRS complex:	Wide complexes Vl–3
	'M' pattern
ST segment:	Depressed Vl–3
T wave:	Inverted Vl–3
U waves:	Absent
Pattern recognition:	(1) RBBB
	(2) Atrial fibrillation, aetiology unknown

Note. ST segment and T wave changes are secondary to RBBB.

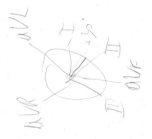

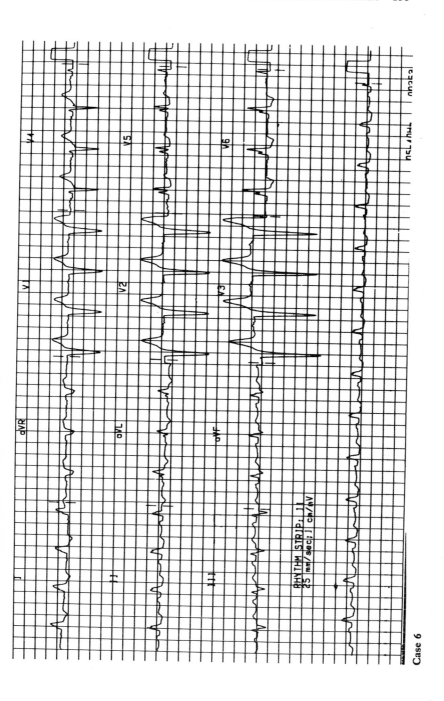

Case 6

Case 6

Rate:	85/min
Rhythm:	Sinus
Axis:	+30°
P wave:	Rather broader than normal
PR interval:	0.16 s
QRS:	Wide
	Bizarre-looking
	'M' pattern V5–6
ST segment:	Depressed I, II, AVF, AVL, V5–6
T waves:	Inverted V5, V6, I, II, AVL
U waves:	Absent
Pattern recognition:	LBBB, aetiology unknown

Note. The ST segment and T wave abnormalities are secondary to
LBBB.

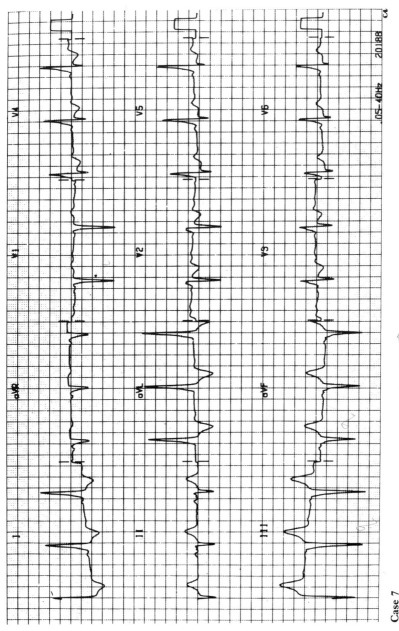

Case 7

Case 7

Rate:	65/min
Rhythm:	Sinus
Axis:	−60° (left axis deviation)
P wave:	Normal
PR interval:	0.1 s (abnormally short)
QRS complex:	Abnormal-looking
	Width 0.12 s
	Slurred upstroke to R wave (delta wave)
ST segment:	Depressed V2–6, I, AVL
T wave:	Inverted V2–4, I, AVL
U waves:	Absent
Pattern recognition:	Wolff–Parkinson–White syndrome

Note. This ECG bears a striking similarity to LBBB (Case 6).

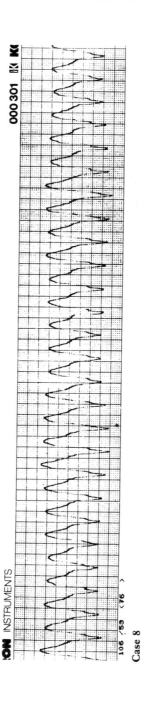

Case 8

Case 8

Broad complex tachycardia.
Rate 150/min.
Diagnosis: ventricular tachycardia (VT).

This may be impossible to distinguish from SVT with aberrant conduction without doing sophisticated electrophysiological studies (see main text).

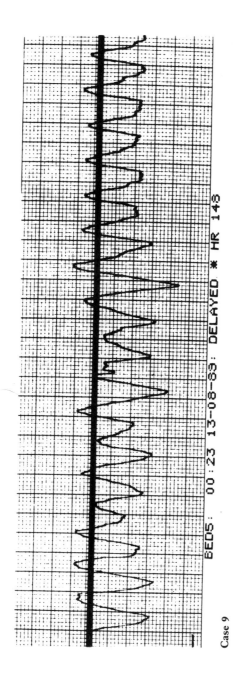

BED5: 00:23 13-08-83: DELAYED * HR 148

Case 9

Case 9

Broad complex trace with no discernible underlying rhythm.
Patient pulseless.
Diagnosis: Ventricular fibrillation (VF).

Call the cardiac arrest team.

KEY QUESTIONS

I have made it easy this time by including the answers.

(1) ECG changes in pulmonary embolus[†]
    none*
    sinus tachycardia[†]
    RBBB[†]
    Sl, Q3, T3[‡] (S wave in I, Q wave in III, inverted T in III).

(2) ECG changes in myocardial infarction[†]
    none
    hyperacute, peaked T waves
    ST elevation
    Q waves
    T wave inversion.

These changes occur over the first 36 hours. Q waves and T wave inversion may persist.

(3) Arrhythmias in myocardial infarction[†]
    The answer to this is easy: any (see earlier).

(4) Causes of sinus bradycardia
    vasovagal syncope
    fit young athletes
    post-myocardial infarction
    iatrogenic (β blocker)
    raised intracranial pressure
    myxoedema
    jaundice
    hypothermia.

(5) Causes of sinus tachycardia
    anxiety
    pain
    post-myocardial infarction
    iatrogenic (β agonists)
    pulmonary embolus
    shock (of any aetiology)
    thyrotoxicosis
    fever.

---

* Very common.
† Common.
‡ Rare and/or difficult.

(6) ECG effects of digoxin
    'reversed tick' sign (Fig. 13.6)
    a-v block
    any arrhythmia, but especially electrical bigeminy and
    paroxysmal atrial tachycardia, with block (digoxin toxicity).

(7) Hypokalaemia[†]
    prominent U wave
    inverted T wave
    ST depression
    PR prolongation (see Fig. 13.7).

(8) Hyperkalaemia[†]
    tall, peaked T wave
    QRS widening
    absent P wave (see Fig. 13.7).

(9) The ECG differences between pericarditis and pericardial effusion:
    pericarditis
        ST elevation (concave upwards) V4–5, I, AVL (Fig. 13.6)
    pericardial effusion
        small-voltage ECG (all leads).

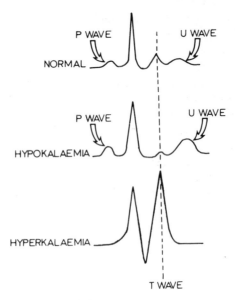

Fig. 13.7 Potassium and the ECG.

(10) The ECG criteria for left ventricular hypertrophy (LVH)
tall R waves V5, 6
deep S waves V1, 2.
Note: If height of R wave in V6 plus depth of S wave in V1
is greater than 40 mm, this is definite evidence of LVH.
inverted T waves (sometimes) V4–6
LAD.

(11) Causes of left axis deviation (LAD)
axis −30° to −120°
left anterior hemiblock
inferior myocardial infarction
chronic obstructive airways disease
Wolff-Parkinson-White syndrome
left ventricular hypertrophy.

(12) Cause of right axis deviation (RAD)
axis + 90° to + 180°
right ventricular hypertrophy
dextrocardia
Wolff-Parkinson-White syndrome
left posterior hemiblock (diagnosed by excluding the others)
leads on wrong way round.

(13) Causes of LBBB
(NB: always an abnormal finding)
ischaemic heart disease
hypertension
aortic valve disease
following cardiac surgery.

(14) Causes of RBBB
pulmonary embolism
ischaemic heart disease
atrial septal defect
chronic pulmonary hypertension
myocarditis
some normal patients.

14 Radiology

The radiographs you may be asked to comment on during the course of the clinical examination or viva will not be complicated or too exotic: this would be unfair.

You need to try to demonstrate several things to the examiner. Firstly, appear as though you are familiar with looking at radiographs. Secondly, show that you have a logical, methodical approach to their interpretation. Finally, demonstrate that you can spot gross abnormalities, even if you are unsure what they represent.

To achieve these aims you need to practise looking at some radiographs, of the kind which crop up in the examination, using a systematic approach to their interpretation.

Approach to the chest radiograph

(1) Always view on a well-lit viewing box

(2) Look at the side marker (L or R)

This is to make sure that the radiograph has been put up the correct way round. There are several causes of a 'R' marker on the left of a chest radiograph:

Radiograph put on the viewing box the wrong way round.
Radiograph marked incorrectly by the radiographer.
Dextrocardia.

In the latter two cases the 'R' marker is on the same side as the cardiac apex.

(3) Check name and date of birth

They may give important clues.

(4) Determine whether the radiograph is a posteroanterior (PA) or anteroposterior (AP)

In PA views the cardiothoracic ratio (ratio of the transverse size of the cardiac outline to the transverse size of the thoracic cage) is normally less than 0.5. An AP projection will cause an apparent increase in this ratio (where none actually exists) because of the way in which the radiograph has been taken. Therefore, you must *never* comment on the cardiothoracic ratio of an AP chest radiograph.

If an AP view has been taken the radiographer should label the film 'AP' (see Case 10). This can be checked by looking at the position of the scapulae on the film. In an AP projection the scapulae overlie the lung fields, but in a good-quality PA view they should not (compare Cases 10 and 11).

(5) View the radiograph as a whole

Your eye may be caught by a gross abnormality.

(6) View each part of the radiograph in turn

Ignore the temptation to blurt out your first impression. You must now methodically look at each part of the radiograph in turn, to see if you can spot any other abnormalities. I use the following scheme:

Soft tissues
  breasts
  subcutaneous tissues
    chest
    neck
    arms.
Bony structures
  humeri
  scapulae
  clavicles
  cervical/thoracic spine
  ribs.
Pleura and diaphragm.
Mediastinal structures.
Lung fields.

(7) Take another look at the radiograph as a whole

(8) Synthesise

Now synthesise the above steps, to arrive at your answer. Remember to relate the radiological findings to any clinical information you already know about the patient.

Try to illustrate to the examiner that you have looked at the radiograph methodically. For example:

Question:	'What abnormalities do you see on this chest radiograph'?
Bad answer: (although correct)	'Carcinoma of the bronchus'.
Good answer:	'There is a 4 cm nodule in the mid-zone of the left lung field. This has a slightly irregular margin. The superior edge is particularly indistinct, with linear shadows radiating into the left upper lobe. The most likely cause for this appearance would be carcinoma of the bronchus. I can see no evidence of metastatic spread to the bones, mediastinal structures or other lung field, which all appear normal'.

This general approach can be applied to any radiograph, including contrast radiology. Once you have got the general idea, all you need is practice.

SPECIMEN CASES

I have included some radiological cases for you to consider. The answers are to be found on the page following each case.

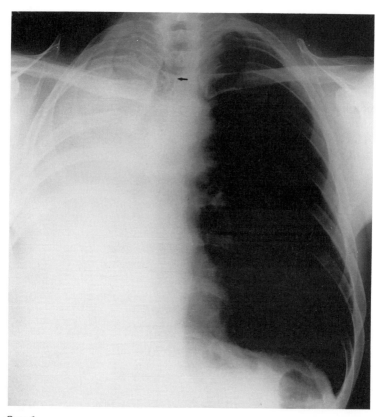

Case 1

Case 1

This is a PA chest radiograph.

The whole of the right lung field is radio-opaque ('white-out').

The arrow indicates the left margin of the trachea. This, together with the position of the cardiac outline (which is barely visible), implies mediastinal shift to the right, due to loss of lung volume on this side.

The right fifth rib is absent.

Soft tissues — normal.

Conclusion. Post-pneumonectomy chest radiograph.

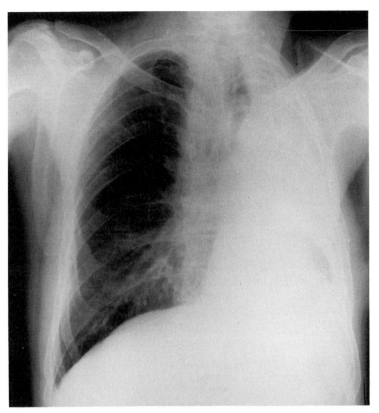

Case 2

Case 2

This is a PA chest radiograph.
The whole of the left lung field is radio-opaque.
There is considerable loss of volume of the left lung (tracheal and mediastinal deviation to the left).
Bony structures — normal.
Soft tissues — normal.

Conclusion. Collapse, left lung. In this case it was due to a large carcinoma of the bronchus obstructing the left main bronchus. This was confirmed at bronchoscopy.

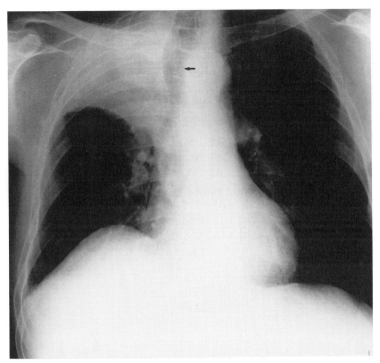

Case 3

Case 3

This is a PA chest radiograph.

The right lung has a homogeneous radio-opaque area in the upper zone. This has a sharply demarcated lower edge, convex upwards, which is almost certainly an abnormally high horizontal fissure.

The trachea is pulled over to the right.

The right hemi-diaphragm is domed medially, and slightly higher than normal.

Bony structures — normal.

Soft tissues — normal.

Conclusion. Partial collapse, right upper lobe.

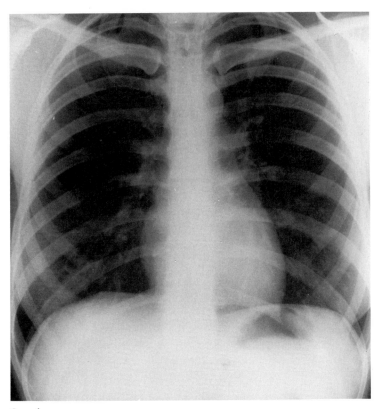

Case 4

Case 4

This is a normal PA chest radiograph.

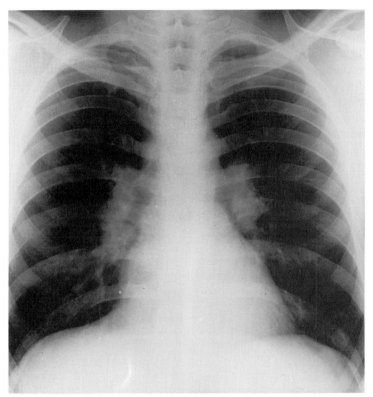

Case 5

Case 5

This is a PA chest radiograph.
There is bilateral hilar lymphadenopathy.
In addition to this there is also paratracheal lymphadenopathy (look adjacent to the trachea, just below the medial end of the right clavicle).
Lung fields — normal.
Pleura — normal.
Bones — normal.
Soft tissues — normal.

Conclusion. Sarcoidosis.

NB: Causes of bilateral hilar lymphadenopathy include:

Sarcoidosis.
Tuberculosis.
Lymphoma.

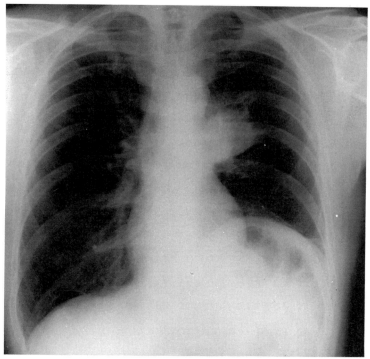

Case 6

Case 6

This is a PA chest radiograph.

There is a mass at the hilum. Its inferior surface is well demarcated, but its superior and lateral edges are irregular. Its medial surface merges with the mediastinal structures.

There is a raised left hemidiaphragm.

Right lung — normal.

Bony structures — normal.

Soft tissues — normal.

Conclusion. Carcinoma of the bronchus causing a left phrenic nerve palsy. The phrenic nerve palsy can be confirmed radiologically by fluoroscopic screening of the diaphragm.

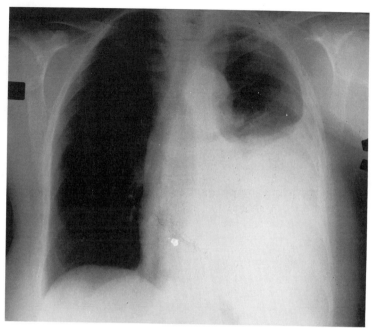

Case 7

Case 7

This is a PA chest radiograph.

There is homogeneous shadowing in the lower and mid-zones of the left lung field. The superior border is well demarcated and concave upwards.

The left costophrenic angle has been obscured.

The mediastinum is central.

The right lung field is normal.

The left breast is absent.

Bony structures — normal.

Conclusion. Left pleural effusion. Subsequent investigation revealed it to be due to metastatic adenocarcinoma. The primary was removed from the left breast 8 years previously.

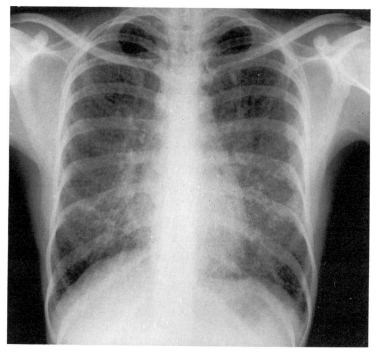

Case 8

Case 8

This is a PA chest radiograph.
There are small nodules (1–2 cm diameter) and fine line shadows spread evenly throughout both lung fields (reticulonodular shadowing). There is, possibly, relative sparing of the apices.
Mediastinal structures — normal.
Pleura/diaphragm — normal.
Bony structures — normal.
Soft tissues — normal.

Conclusion. Reticulonodular shadowing, cause unknown. There are many possible causes, including:

Miliary tuberculosis.
Sarcoidosis.
Pneumoconiosis.
Lymphangitis carcinomatosa.

Case 8 was due to sarcoidosis.

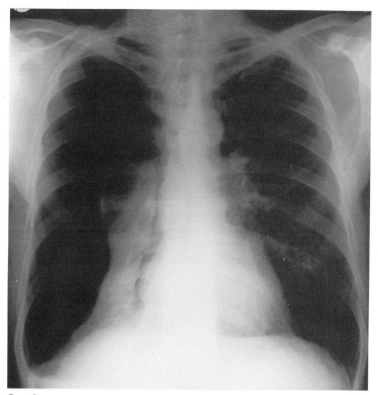

Case 9

Case 9

Conclusion. Large right pneumothorax.

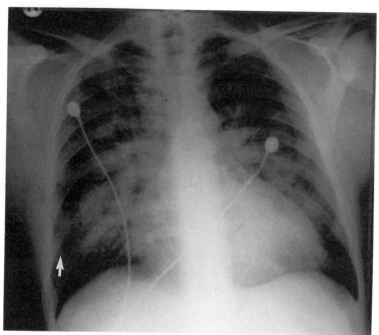

Case 10

Case 10

This is a AP chest radiograph. Note the position of the medial border of the scapulae, which commonly project over the edge of the lung fields in an AP film.

There is fluffy shadowing in both lung fields, particularly in the mid-zones. The upper lobe vessels are bulky.

There are Kerley B lines (arrowed at the right base).

Soft tissues — normal.

Pleura and diaphragm — normal.

Bony structures — normal.

Conclusion. Pulmonary oedema.

NB: You cannot comment on the cardiac size on this film, even though it looks large, as it is an AP view.

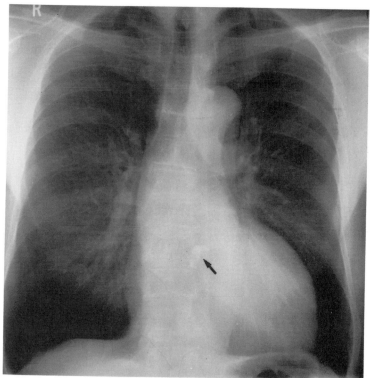

Case 11

Case 11

This is a PA chest radiograph.

The cardiothoracic ratio is 0.52, which is just above the normal limit. There is an area of calcification overlying the cardiac silhouette (arrowed). This represents a calcified aortic valve, although it is impossible to say this with certainty without doing a lateral view.

The lung fields contain a generalised increase in vascular markings, and in particular the upper lobe blood vessels look bulky.

Soft tissues — normal.

Pleura and diaphragm — normal.

Bony structures — normal.

Conclusion. Calcific aortic stenosis, with secondary increase in pulmonary venous pressure.

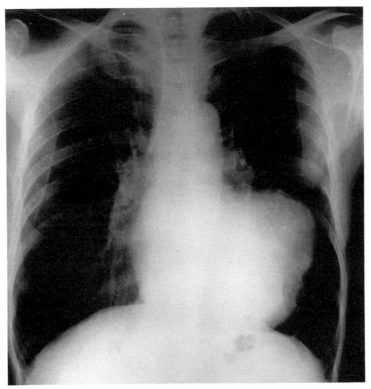

Case 12

Case 12

This is a PA chest radiograph.

Cardiothoracic ratio = 0.56 (abnormal).

There is cardiomegaly. The main area of cardiac enlargement is on the left side of the cardiac outline, which also appears to have a double shadow. The left border of the heart is considerably 'bowed-out' (convex outwards).

Lung fields — normal.

Soft tissues — normal.

Pleura and diaphragm — normal.

Bony structures — normal.

Conclusion. Left ventricular enlargement due to a cardiac aneurysm.

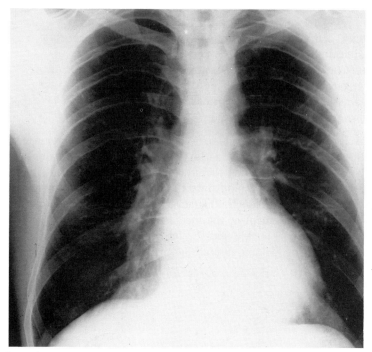

Case 13

Case 13

This is a PA chest radiograph.
Mediastinum — normal.
Lung fields — normal.
Soft tissues — normal.
Pleura and diaphragm — normal.
Bony structures — abnormal.

Conclusion. This radiograph demonstrates classical rib notching, as found in coarctation of the aorta. This is seen on the inferior surfaces of the ribs, overlying the mid-zones of both lung fields. This radiograph does not demonstrate the other radiological feature of coarctation — post-stenotic dilatation of the aorta. This would be seen as an enlargement of the mediastinal shadow in the area between the aortic knuckle and the left hilum. This case illustrates the necessity of looking carefully and methodically at all areas of the radiograph.

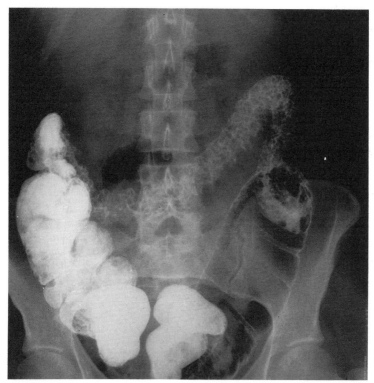

Case 14

Case 14

This is a barium enema examination.

The transverse colon shows a grossly abnormal appearance. Throughout the whole of the transverse and proximal descending colon there is severe and continuous mucosal ulceration and oedema. There is loss of the normal haustral pattern in this region. The abnormalities show relative sparing of the ascending colon.

Conclusion. These findings are in keeping with the diagnosis of ulcerative colitis.

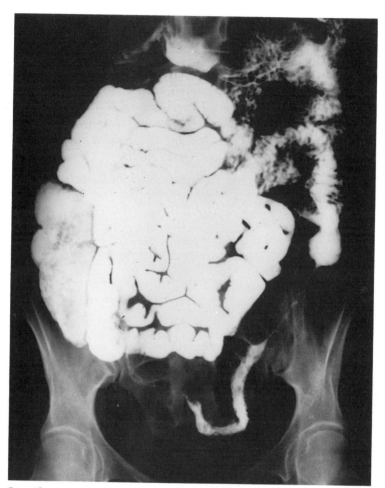

Case 15

Case 15

This is a small bowel contrast study.

Barium outlines the small bowel. In addition there is a small amount of contrast in the stomach and duodenal cap (top of the picture).

There is an area of stricturing of the small bowel (overlying the left sacroiliac joint). Proximal to this there is a short length of bowel with abnormal mucosa. This demonstrates mucosal oedema and ulceration, including several 'rose-thorn' ulcers.

Conclusion. These findings are compatible with Crohn's disease.

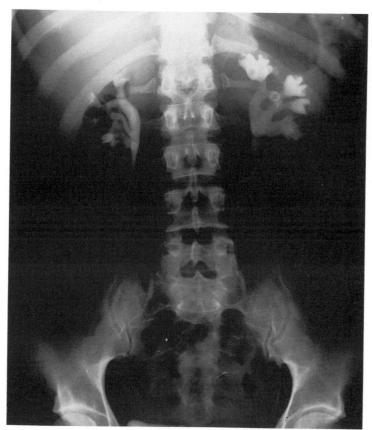

Case 16a

Case 16a

This is an intravenous urogram (IVU).

Contrast is seen in both pelvicalyceal systems and proximal ureters. The left ureter can just be seen in the pelvis.

The left pelvicalyceal system is slightly dilated, compared with the right. However the diameter of the ureter on the left appears normal.

Bladder — not seen.

Bony structures — normal.

Soft tissues — normal.

Conclusion. Slight enlargement of the left pelvicalyceal system, cause unknown.

If you are asked to comment on an IVU always ask to see a control film (a plain radiograph, before contrast was given). Please see Case 16b.

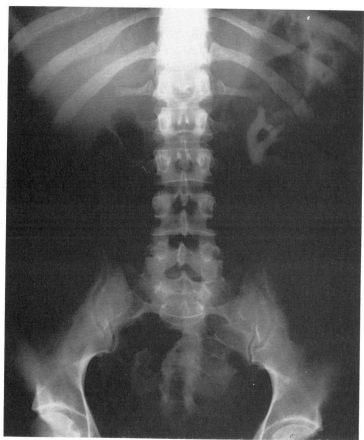

Case 16b

Case 16b

This is a control film for the IVU shown in Case 16a, and was therefore taken before the injection of contrast.
The cause of the minimal dilatation of the left pelvicalyceal system is now obvious. There is a large staghorn calculus on the left.

Note. It is impossible to make this diagnosis from the IVU alone, without seeing the control film.

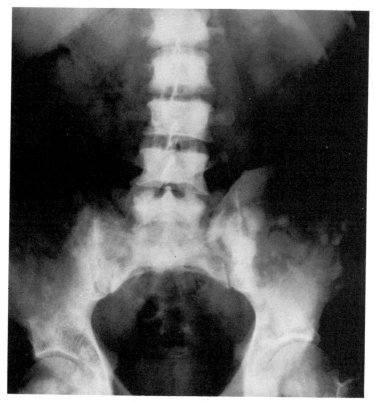

Case 17

Case 17

This is a plain radiograph of the pelvis.
There are sclerotic deposits throughout the lumbar spine and pelvis.

Conclusion. This appearance is seen in carcinoma of: prostate
breast
thyroid.

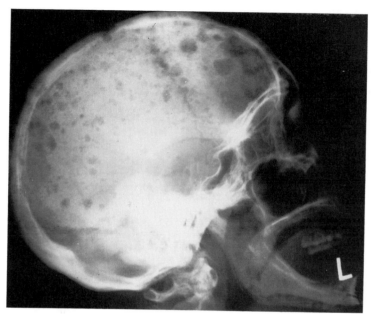

Case 18

Case 18

This is a lateral skull radiograph.
There are multiple circular defects of varying sizes throughout the vault of the skull. These also affect the mandible.

Conclusion. This is a characteristic appearance of multiple myeloma.

NB: Causes of 'holes' in the vault of the skull include:

Congenital.
Malignant tumours
   myeloma
   metastatic carcinoma
   lymphoma.
Benign tumours
   neurofibroma.
Arteriovenous malformations.

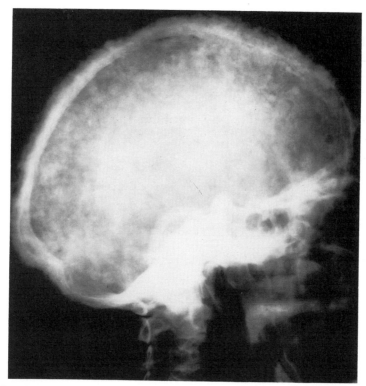

Case 19

Case 19

This is a lateral skull radiograph.
There are multiple, fluffy opacities throughout the skull.

Conclusion. This 'cotton wool' effect is characteristic of Paget's disease.

Index

Page numbers in bold type refer to headings in text.

Weber test, 96, 97
Wegener's granulomatosis, 132
Weil's disease, 60
Wernicke's area, 98
Wickham's striae, 80
Wilson's disease, 58, 113

Wolff-Parkinson-White syndrome,
141, 142, 157, 158, 165

Xanthelasmata, 34, 70, 87, 132

Z-deformity, thumb, 121